WRECKED

WHY YOUR QUEST FOR HEALTH AND WEIGHT LOSS
HAS FAILED AND WHAT YOU CAN DO ABOUT IT

DR. STEVE PRENTICE

Publishing services provided by:

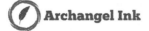 Archangel Ink

ISBN-13: 978-1545504369
ISBN: 1545504369

Contents

Part I

WRECKED

I've tried everything . . . and I'm just getting worse.

I've done everything they told me to do but nothing works.

I feel like my body is defective.

I feel like I'm banging my head against a wall.

I'm so sick of thinking about weight and health.

If I read another diet book I'm going to throw up in my mouth!

Unfortunately, these are the thoughts, feelings, and experiences that millions of people live with every day. I'd imagine that because you are reading a book called *Wrecked: Why Your Quest for Health and Weight Loss Has Failed—and What You Can Do about It,* maybe you can relate to the above sentiments.

Whether it's a desire to lose weight, a wish to get fit, an attempt to regain lost health, or a need to prevent future problems, you no doubt have had experience in attempting to implement ideas presented to you by a health authority (or someone claiming to be one). Endless diets, eating philosophies, exercise programs, and supplementation regimens abound, almost always resulting in a failure to deliver promised results.

The hope ending in disappointment, the repeat wasted

efforts, the exhausting, constant exertion of willpower (only to end in failure), and the endless frustration of being at war with your body can sap the joy out of life. And if that's not enough, they can (and usually *will*) further damage the very health you're trying so desperately to improve.

My intention is that, by the end of this book, you will have a renewed sense of hope. A hope based in reality and reason, and not on a false narrative that implies if you would just work hard enough and straighten yourself up that you too could achieve all your health and wellness dreams.

I want you to appreciate what you're *really* up against so that you can direct your focus appropriately and have an actual shot at succeeding.

Most of all, I want you to get off the Tilt-A-Whirl of futility, get your life back, and stop with the self-abuse masquerading as "improving my health." In other words—and I can't believe I am saying this—you need to check yourself before you wreck yourself.

This is *not* another weight loss book. You won't have to go shopping to restock your cupboards full of obscure food or cancel any and all holidays with family because your diet is so rigid and joyless that you can't even have a meal with other people. In fact, my goal is that by implementing what you learn in this book, you will think about food *less than you ever have before*.

Can (or will) you lose weight following my recommendations? Depends on what you mean by "lose weight." If you're looking to temporarily lose twenty pounds by next Tuesday, then no. However, if you're interested in effortlessly and legitimately dropping some body fat over time by getting your life back and setting yourself free from health and diet nonsense, *then I may have your answer.*

This book is about freedom—freedom to live your life without obsessing about health and weight. Freedom to live your life without obsessing about basic body functions such as eating, drinking, sleeping, and using the bathroom, and the *damage that results* from *obsessing about* eating, drinking, sleeping, and using the bathroom. Freedom to live at peace with your biology. Freedom to be as healthy as you can be with very little effort. Freedom from living under the tyranny of unrealistic expectations. Freedom to live like a normal person. And maybe best of all, freedom from paying any more attention to health and diet gurus (priceless).

*****

This is what I call a "get-to-the-point" book.

Being an avid reader for most of my life, I have come to the conclusion that most books (non-fiction) are entirely too long. I don't know about you but I read non-fiction because I want to learn something. I appreciate longer novels because they're designed to be enjoyed while relaxing, so the longer the better, assuming they're entertaining. Non-fiction, though, is different. I would much rather learn something in three hours than in three days. I've got a life to lead and a Facebook wall to monitor, after all.

On average, I would say the ideas contained in most non-fiction books could be condensed down to sixty pages or so, which is usually plenty to get the points across. Everything else is just fluff and filler used to extend the length, give the perception of increased value, and to justify being called a "book." Well nuts to that! I say we skip the nonsense and just get to the point.

This book is meant to be like a hostage rescue. You get in, get what you need, and get out. Therefore, I've cut it down to the minimum length while still making all of my points. I guess if you really want a longer book you can just read it twice. A lot of what you're going to read comes from my own personal experience and observation working with patients as a practicing chiropractor for twenty years, my own conclusions from twenty years of researching the latest and greatest in health enhancement and recovery, learning from mentors that know more than me, and of course, scientific literature.

A word about "science" though. Science is great and wonderful. It allows us the ability to uncover the secrets of the universe and unlock the mysteries of life and all that stuff. It's also as corrupt, political, and flawed as the day is long. While the purpose of this book is not a critique of the science "industry," please understand the reality that science (especially health science) is an agenda and money-driven game rife with fraud just like everything else. Write a check big enough and you can get a study to say anything you want. Manipulate statistics and data and you can get virtually any outcome you want. So while I value a well-designed, agenda-free study as much as anybody, I don't worship at the altar of the laboratory and I don't suspend all critical thinking.

I also don't need a randomized, triple-blind, controlled clinical trial to tell me the obvious. Some science worshippers I know take it to the extreme and need *everything* confirmed with an experiment. I think that's narrow-minded and silly. So while of course science is an important tool when it comes to the human body, I don't need a published study in a peer-reviewed journal to convince me that I do, in fact, need to pee when I get up in the morning.

Research is often used as a manipulation tool as opposed to a tool to satisfy a genuine desire for knowledge. My experience has been that people demanding studies to validate your point are rarely ever satisfied with what you produce. They also tend to have a *much* higher standard of proof required for opinions with which they don't agree. Oftentimes, people buy into a story and then cherry-pick studies to back up their assertion. I am hopeful the conclusions I draw in this book will be fairly self-evident. If not, I guess you can just keep doing what you're doing.

That being said, I've decided to leave the references out of the book except for when I'm quoting someone else's work.

Just a couple of ground rules before we get rolling.

Try to digest the ideas in this book with an open mind. Don't be too sensitive. Being offended is a tremendous waste of time and energy so let your guard down and don't take anything too personally. I'll probably write something at some point that pokes you. I'm snarky like that. Don't tighten up on me. Unclench the cheeks and roll with it. For instance, a *lot* of people have based their entire identities on what they eat and how they exercise so simply questioning the logic of some diet practices are to them, fightin' words. If this describes you, please realize you are not your food. And if you get insulted by a remark about a diet, then I suggest it's a *neon-red flag* that you need to read this book slowly and maybe even more than once.

I will also be discussing behavior and personality issues that come into play with the topic of health and health obsession and some may hit home. It's okay. I'm just asking that you do a little honest self-examination and consider my points.

Lastly, I may question a conclusion or belief you hold near and dear. That's okay too. Dig your heels in if you wish, but at least consider the point.

So to sum up—don't be offended, be open-minded, be willing to examine your beliefs and behaviors, and be willing to consider my points.

At its essence, this is a book written by a health professional who's trying to convince you to chill out with the health thing and drastically reduce your health improvement efforts. Yes, I know it sounds strange and a little ironic but the reality is there's a lot at stake—namely your health, happiness, and quality of life.

As a practicing chiropractor working with thousands of patients for the last twenty years, I've observed (and experienced firsthand) a puzzling phenomenon—oftentimes, the more we do to improve our health, the worse it gets.

Is this 100 percent of the time? No, but it's *very* common.

In fact, it's becoming more and more common the more health obsessed we become as a society and the motivation to write this book stemmed from watching the health and quality of life of too many people be destroyed by adopting health practices that, while sounding good, actually caused harm.

Isn't it ironic that one of the biggest threats to your health is your attempt to get healthy?

In practicing over the years, I've also noticed that patients tend to fall into one of three groups:

1. Those with symptoms resulting from the effects of accumulated stress
2. Those with symptoms of accumulated stress + the negative effects of their attempts to fix it
3. Those that were hit by a truck (or other trauma)

Stress or trauma. That about sums it up.

It doesn't matter what condition, what kind of doctor, or what symptom, it's either going to be caused by accumulated stress or the result of a trauma. I don't want to get bogged down too long on this point (that's for the next book) but I want you to appreciate this point because I'm giving you a "golden nugget."

When it comes to health, stress is everything.

No, really. It's all about stress. This is where all health care practitioners, medical and non-medical, would be in agreement. Boil it all down and what you end up with is that stress is hands down the number one cause of health problems—and there's not a close second.

If you think about it, even trauma is nothing more than a physical stress that overwhelms the body's ability to adapt, resulting in damage. If you fall off the second rung of a ladder, that is a physical stress your body can absorb without tissue damage. Fall off the tenth rung and it's a different story. It's a higher level of physical stress capable of snapping your femur. So even trauma can be included in the statement "stress is everything."

For the sake of our discussion, however, let's put aside physical trauma when we talk about stress and health because that's by *far* the smallest group that ends up in doctors' offices (even though most people think it's the biggest).

The other two types of stress besides physical are chemical (including environmental) and emotional (which includes psychological and spiritual). Both chemical and environmental stresses include anything that goes in or on your body that cause a stress response. Emotional stress is the stuff that goes on in your head.

So we have physical, chemical, and emotional stress. If your body can adapt to and handle these stresses successfully and efficiently, then everything functions normally and you are "healthy." If your body is over-whelmed by any of these stresses, then dysfunction and "dis-*ease*" will result. If this dysfunction and dis-ease is allowed to remain long enough, then eventually you will start showing signs and symptoms, and based on how those signs show up, you will be given a diagnosis. Dis-ease eventually leads to disease.

I often use the analogy of a bicycle tire to describe stress and our bodies. A certain amount of air is required for a bike tire to be effective and useful. If the tire is underinflated, then it is "flat" and utterly useless. If it is overinflated, then it will still function but the risk is high that it will eventually blow out.

In the human body, stress is a neurological phenomenon. Stress is perceived and experienced in your nervous system, and it's your nervous system that is responsible for "processing" the stress as it occurs.

So think of your nervous system as the bike tire. If there was *no* stress getting "pumped in" or experienced, that would not be good. We need a certain level of stress to get us out of bed in the morning! The right amount and type of stress can be healthy and productive. If there is too much stress getting pumped in, however, the nervous system becomes "overinflated."

A stressed-out nervous system is not good, because it's your nervous system that runs everything in your body. A distressed nervous system by definition means the body cannot and will not function normally.

An "overinflated" or overstressed nervous system may manifest as sleep disturbances, digestive issues, headaches, anxiety, depression, aches, pains, and metabolic changes, for example. You may still function at some level but the red flags are waving, indicating the system is overtaxed.

If those signs are ignored and more stress is pumped in, then there is a serious danger of a blowout. A stress blowout can be a heart attack, stroke, emotional or psychological breakdown, autoimmune disorders, cancer, or any myriad of ways the body hits the wall.

So if the body can process out the stress faster than you pump it in, you'll be okay. If your body cannot process the stress faster than you pump it in, then the stress accumulates, and eventually you'll be overinflated and, worst case scenario, you'll have a blowout.

Pretty simple, right? That's why I describe group 1 as "those with symptoms resulting from the effects of accumulated stress." That pretty much describes everyone in any doctor's office anywhere.

Group 2 is for the most part just like group 1, but with an added wrinkle. Before group 2 shows up to our office they have researched and tried things on their own to remedy their situation. Is that bad? Not necessarily. I think it would be a little strange and childish if people ran to the doctor for every single minor twinge or tingle. And with the advent of the "Google machine," I think it's perfectly reasonable to research what's bothering you on your own. So it's not that group 2 did something bad or inappropriate. Where it goes wrong is that they are usually given bad advice.

Group 2 has grown exponentially in the last few years. It goes something like this:

- » Person experiences stress
- » Stress accumulates over months and years
- » Body eventually starts showing signs
- » Signs get more and more uncomfortable or unacceptable
- » Person seeks answers as to how to reverse signs
- » Person tries what they have learned (usually diet/exercise changes)
- » Person eventually fails and/or gets worse
- » Person tries something else
- » Person eventually fails and/or gets worse

- » Rinse and repeat for years or decades
- » Person now worse than ever
- » Person ends up wishing they had never tried anything
- » Person hopelessly confused

So group 2 has the signs/symptoms of accumulated stress (like group 1) but now they also have issues caused by whatever stress/damage was added by their attempt to fix it.

It's like if my kitchen sink were to spring a leak. I would consider calling a plumber, but then discouraged by the hassle and cost, try to fix it myself. My attempt would go horribly awry (because I'm useless with tools), and then I would have to call the plumber to fix the original leak *plus* the cracked pipe, stripped threads, and broken clamp from my attempt.

Before we move on, we need to discuss a subgroup under group 2.

Group 2 as I have described it is simply people that started having some kind of health issue and then researched possible fixes on their own and started trying remedies, resulting in additional problems. That used to make up most of the group 2s. In the last few years, however, another path has evolved that also leads to group 2. We'll call this group 2b.

What makes group 2b different is that they ended up there not necessarily because of an actual health issue but because of

>> A fear of a future health issue

>> Attempts to lose weight

>> A desire to become "optimum"

>> Vanity

So let's take a moment and delve a little further into the 2bs (pronounced toobies).

Generation Selfie

I blame most of society's problems on Facebook. No, really.

It was launched in 2004 but from my perception it really started making its impact around 2009. It was then that it seemed to transition from being a teenager/college-kid thing to the all-ages phenomenon it is today. Indeed, 2009 was when we all began to feast on the minutiae of each other's lives.

Seemingly overnight we became a country of narcissistic nightmares. Many acquaintances I assumed were reasonably well-adjusted revealed themselves via social media to be self-obsessed, angst-filled teenagers trapped in middle-aged adult bodies.

What started as a way to keep up with our close friends and family turned into a daily log of the mundane: A photo of what I ate for breakfast. A photo of my Starbucks cup. A summary of my trip to the grocery store. A photo of the grocery store. A selfie of me in the produce aisle. A photo of a cloud. A summary of my workout. A photo of the gym. The course I walked through the neighborhood. A sweaty selfie of me after my workout. A photo of my lunch.

Another selfie (with duck lips). A photo of my feet while sitting in a chaise lounge. A photo of my glass of wine. A post about how my life is so great. A selfie of me in a mirror taking a selfie. A photo of dinner. A post about how my relationship is so great. A cryptic post that no one understands but implies something bad is happening. Another selfie. A post about how tired I am. A photo of the banana I'm eating. A post about how underappreciated I am. Another selfie. A post about what movie I'm watching. A philosophical meme. A good-night selfie.

Then get up the next day and do it again until 892 of your 920 "friends" have blocked you.

This begs the chicken-or-the-egg question, "Did Facebook cause the narcissism or did it simply allow the already narcissistic a forum to spread their wings and fly?"

Who knows, probably both, but this extreme focus on the self has spilled over into the health realm. Now obviously Facebook (and social media in general) is but one factor that has contributed to the reality of today, but it's this obsession of the self that is at the core of the problem. Add to that the ability to compare ourselves to hundreds of people in real time and you have the makings of a mess.

Am I happy enough? Do I have enough friends? Do I have as much fun as them? Am I as fulfilled? Do I eat more than them? Do I exercise enough? Am I bigger? Am I smaller? Do I have enough bowel movements? Do I eat too many carbs? Do I eat enough kale? Should I drink more smoothies? Am I fit enough? Should I be able to run farther? Should my kids be acting different? Should my skin look better? Should I sleep better? Should I look better? Should I be healthier? Am I too lazy? Should I be tanner? Should I have more money? Should I be more spiritual? Should I be peeing more? Should my urine be clear? Do I drink enough water? And on and on and on into a bottomless pit of self-examination, self-criticism, and comparison to others.

The result? You *always* fall short.

You could be/should be:

» Skinnier

» More fit

» Better looking

» Happier

» More fulfilled

- » More successful
- » Healthier
- » Younger looking
- » More accomplished
- » Eating better
- » Exercising more
- » A better mom
- » A better dad
- » Et cetera

You can (and should) *be* it all and *have* it all. In fact, the *entire point* of living is self-improvement!

Do you realize how much you're missing out on? Just look at your friends. See how great their lives are? See how good they look? See how popular they are? You could have it all too if you'd just put out the effort! What's wrong with you?

Is it any wonder everyone's depressed?

So the noble-on-the-surface quest for optimum begins, and usually starts with the quest for optimum health and weight. What's wrong with that? Isn't it a good thing to strive to be the best *you* possible? Isn't it a good thing to try and clean up your act? To improve your lifestyle? Well, sure, to a degree.

The reality, however, is all too commonly something different.

To be fair, it's not all narcissistic-driven behavior that leads people to chase the unicorn of optimum health ("optimum" doesn't really exist because you can always improve, theoretically). Are some motivated to take action to improve their health because of legitimate diseases, conditions, and/or injuries, and not some obsessive desire to achieve the imagined ecstasy of perfection? Of course! Be careful, though, the person legitimately seeking to regain their lost health, well-being, and ability to function is just as vulnerable to digging their hole deeper as is the fitness fanatic who thinks life will become magical if they can just push that truck tire over one more time.

Health is great. We all want it and that's okay. In the last few years, however, something has changed. A shift has taken place in the psyche of Americans. Health has gone from something that allows us to *fulfill* our purpose in life to *being* the purpose in life. In other words, being healthy is necessary for life but it shouldn't be the *point* of life. If you were the healthiest specimen ever to walk the Earth, yet you just sat in a room and stared at a wall for ninety years, I would suggest that your life would be an *epic fail*. Being some kind of supreme health specimen is pointless in and of itself.

When health goes from being a means to an end *to the actual end* is when it becomes unhealthy. It's like having a car. The value of a car is that it enables you to travel long distances quickly, which in turn enables you to accomplish more in life. So a car is indeed a valuable tool in life! In fact, it is so valuable that we go to great expense and effort to make sure the car runs well and is dependable because, after all, a broken down car is quite useless. Realize that the value of the car is in what it enables you to accomplish. The value is not just in the fact that it runs well. If your car runs great but all you do is drive it back and forth to the mechanic and gas station to ensure it keeps running well, then it really serves no useful purpose.

You do what you need to do to keep it running and then get on with the important things the car allows you to accomplish. You do your basic maintenance and get on with life. You don't obsess about all the different parts and whether they could be running a little bit "better" if you could only find the secrets to squeezing out a little more performance.

In other words, too many people have an *unhealthy* obsession with *health*.

The Perfect Storm

Looking back over the last twenty years, I can state that the health status of new patients presenting to our office is getting worse and worse. Addiction rates are skyrocketing. Anxiety and depression are at all-time highs. Sleep difficulties, fatigue, headaches, and immune system disorders are commonplace. Normal digestion is getting increasingly rare. Everyone's hypothyroid. Blood sugar abnormalities are routine. Adrenals are exhausted. Food sensitivities are becoming the norm.

These issues individually are hardly a new phenomenon but to see *all* of them seem to go off the charts in the last ten years or so has begged the question, "What the heck is going on?"

I believe there are a number of factors that have coalesced to flush the collective health of Americans down the proverbial toilet.

Stress levels are sky high

As we discussed earlier, the accumulated effects of stress are largely responsible for the dysfunction and dis-ease in the body, leading to health problems. I don't think it's a coincidence that we are seeing a decline in health at the same time we're witnessing an increase in stress and stress-related illnesses.

I was born in 1970 and, in my youth in the '70s and '80s, about the biggest thing we had to worry about was getting nuked by the Russians. I distinctly remember the nuclear bomb drills in which we would crawl under our desks at school. What a plan. I guess the thinking was that the petrified gum stuck under the desktops would somehow soak up the radiation and that the sturdy design would protect us from the blast. Anyway, while Russian nukes were technically considered a threat I don't know if any us were too concerned about it actually happening.

Fast-forward thirty-five years to 2016. The economy is in shambles. The debt is beyond comprehension. Social Security and Medicare are on life support. We don't know if we'll have a job next week, month, or year. We don't know how our kids are going to be able to make a living. The government is out of control and unresponsive. The family unit is disintegrating. Addiction is skyrocketing. States and cities are going bankrupt. Constant wars. Terrorism. School shootings and massacres are on the rise. Twenty-four-hour-a-day news cycles with nothing but politicians arguing. A never-ending barrage of protests, fighting, violence, and crisis. Need I go on? It seems that every foundation our society has been built on is crumbling beneath our feet. And as bad as it is for someone my age to see the foundations crumble, think of the younger generation that *never experienced them in the first place.* Add to this the social degeneration, the decline of face-to-face relationships and friendships, the disconnection from God, and what do we end up with?

A world that seemingly has gone off the rails, with angst and fear being the order of the day. Or is it just me?

So if stress levels are through the roof, it stands to reason that stress-related health challenges are sure to follow. In fact, I *rarely* have a patient that doesn't report stress is a real problem for them. It's almost universal at this point.

Many of the do-it-yourself cures are backfiring

The second factor in the storm is the inadvertently piling on of *additional* stress during the attempt to improve our lifestyles. Whether it's someone trying to clean up their act in an attempt to overcome a health concern, changing their diet in the hope of losing weight, or an already healthy person seeking to achieve "optimum" superhuman status, the current recommendations floating around the Internet and health circles often result in adding gas to the already raging stress fire.

We're going to cover these recommendations momentarily but for now let me just make the point that many of the new school health practices are simply adding more stress to an already overstressed organism (that's you). Whether it's detoxing, cleansing, restrictive dieting, over-exercising, or over-hydrating, the hallmark of today's enlightened health approach is to go to extremes. Everything is hardcore. Why is it that the health practices that promise to bring you to the glorious land of health, vibrancy, and immortality *always* involve lifestyle changes that only the most hardcore, OCD, masochistic, and pathologically driven can achieve?

This is the trap. According to the new school, the price to pay to regain and/or reach "optimum" health is for you to become an obsessive, monomaniacal samurai of self-denial, which in turn requires feats of will that turn you into an obsessive, self-absorbed hot mess.

If the primary factor in determining the health status of an individual is both the level of accumulated stress and the body's available reserves to handle it effectively, then how is piling on a dump truck full of psychological, emotional, *and* physical stress by requiring Evel Knievel levels of difficult and dangerous health stunts supposed to help?

"Ladies and gentlemen! I'm Vern Gabelson and today we will witness local elementary school teacher Sally Knievel attempt a fourteen-day okra juice cleanse all so she can 'look cuter in yoga pants' and add a little more pep in her step! How do you feel, Sally?"

"I feel good," she says apprehensively. "I need to do this . . ."

"What drove you to want to take on this incredible feat of health, dedication, and commitment, Sally?"

"Well, it seems like everyone else is doing it and I've been reading about these cleanses on the Internet for a long time now. In fact, my neighbor Tina is on day eight of a gluten-free, casein-free, nightshade vegetable-free, meat-free, grain-free, sugar-free, fat-free, carb-free, yeast-free, taste-free, joy-free, low acid, raw-only, intermittent fasting cleanse, and I felt like

I was missing out. Well, that, and I don't ever want to die."

"Wow! Tina sounds like she's going to have some awesome selfies soon! How is she doing?"

"Well," Sally replies, "I'm not really sure. Now that you mention it I haven't seen her come out of her house in a couple of days."

"Well I'm sure she's thriving. Are you ready?!"

"Absolutely! Let's do this!"

"Okay, folks, we're ready to go! Sally is stepping up to the counter. She's eyeing the juicer. She has a look of stern resolve—she wants this! She's dropping the okra into the basket. She's placing the lid on. She's turned it on! The juicer is juicing, folks! The juice is coming out! It is *bright* green and it ... it ... wow, what's that smell?"

"That's the smell of vibrant health, Vern! The smell of awesomeness!"

"The glass of juice is about full. Okay, she's turned off the juicer. She has the glass. How do you feel, Sally? Are you going to sip or just down the whole twenty ounces?"

"Down the hatch, Vern."

"Godspeed, Sally! She's doing it! She's drinking the okra juice! She's gulping it down like nectar from the gods! She's almost done! A little more, Sally! She's done it! She finished the entire twenty ounces in one fantastic guzzle! How do you feel, Sally?! How did it taste?!"

"Oh, um,"—*burp*—"it was delicious"—*gurgle*—"almost *too* sweet"—*eeeeyyyuaaaaaaggchch* . . .

"Oh no! Sally just lurched and vomited all over the juicer! This is a disaster! Oh the smell! Sally, are you okay?"

"I think I'm okay," Sally says, picking her head up out of the juicer and wiping green smudge off her forehead. "I must be detoxing."

"Well hang in there, Sally. You only have thirteen-plus days to go."

"Thanks, Vern. And thanks to all the view . . . er . . . I have to go to the bathroom . . ."

Okay, I'll stop. I could seriously keep this going for twenty more pages but let's move on for now.

The "cures" are worse than the disease

Once the accumulated stress rises to the point of a health problem and the Internet and neighbor recommended attempts to fix it have piled on, it's then time to go to the doctor.

From my perspective the practice of being a general practitioner or "family doctor" has been whittled down to essentially handing out prescriptions for antidepressants, antibiotics, statins, ADHD meds for the kids, and painkillers. Better health through chemistry is alive and well. And while youngsters getting into medicine may dream of using their newfound knowledge and insight to lead the masses to the glorious oasis of health, the reality hits home quickly that flowchart medicine is the model of the day:

Symptom X ➜ Drug A

Symptom Y ➜ Drug B

Lab finding Z ➜ Drug C

And by the way, the flowcharts were conveniently created by the pharmaceutical companies, which is why all flowcharts lead to drugs.

In a related story, WebMD reported in 2015 that

burnout rates are soaring for family doctors with 50 percent of *all* family doctors reporting feeling burned out.

But while the doctor business may be losing its luster, the prescription pad business is booming! Researchers from the Mayo Clinic reported in 2013 that 70 percent of *all* Americans are on at least one prescription drug and more than half are on two or more. Twenty percent of Americans are on five or more.

Now listen up. The second largest number of prescriptions was for antidepressants and they report that 13 percent of *all* Americans are on them. Now *that's* depressing.

It gets better. The third largest number of prescriptions was for opioids and they were the most common prescription among young and middle-aged adults.

All I can say to this is *thank you, doctors!* We have an epidemic of opiate addiction in this country that typically starts out with prescribed painkillers such as Percocet, Vicodin, and OxyContin, and then progresses to heroin. Drug overdoses are now the leading cause of injury-related deaths.

Injury-related deaths per year

Drug overdose: 44,000

Motor vehicle deaths: 33,000

Homicide: 16,000

I can't tell you how often new patients that have been prescribed these narcotics for relatively minor to moderate pain come in to our office. My wife Susan is active in our community's recovery movement and we can tell you firsthand that the number of lives and families that have been utterly destroyed by these drugs is alarming and tragic. But it's not just the pain-killers that are causing the pain.

According to Harvard University, in 2014 side effects to *properly prescribed* drugs killed 128,000 people (this does *not* include mistakes) and 1.9 million were hospitalized because of side effects. So side effects to prescription drugs are the fourth leading cause of *death* in the United States only behind heart disease (611,000), cancer (585,000), and respiratory disease (149,000).

So add the 128,000 deaths and the 1.9 million hospitalizations and we have over 2 *million* people that are either hospitalized or dead from properly prescribed drugs. Please realize that these numbers are just for the dead and/or hospitalized. If we add to this the people that were permanently harmed but *weren't* hospitalized, the numbers get even more ridiculous. Add to that the people who were harmed and don't know it (asymptomatic damage) and it gets even crazier. So it would be safe to say that several million people a year are harmed by prescription drugs—oh wait, I forgot to include the over-the-counter drugs numbers! Better get the calculator . . .

Don't misunderstand. I'm not suggesting that medication is never appropriate. My point is that medication should be a *last resort*, not a first line of defense. I haven't met too many people who were on multiple prescription medications that I would consider "healthy." It's actually quite the opposite.

So to sum up the formula as to why the health and quality of life of Americans seems to be in freefall:

» Stress levels are intensifying +
» Attempts to self-correct are making it worse +
» Doctors relying almost exclusively on drugs that are risky and rarely addressing cause
» = Toilet water health

Whether you reached this place because of attempts to solve your stress-induced health issues or because you inadvertently caused the problems yourself on a Don Quixote-like pursuit of awesomeness and rock-hard abs, once your health has reached toilet water status, everything will snowball because you'll be on the constant lookout for solutions. It becomes like quicksand in that the harder you try to get out the faster you sink.

At this point I've hopefully laid the groundwork for us to move forward with our discussion. In the coming chapters we'll cover diet, weight loss, and exercise, and I'll give you a great list of action steps to help you move forward in your quest to regain your health (and sanity).

Each topic above could be a book in and of itself but the purpose of this book is not to be an exhaustive tome on these subjects. Again, this is a get-to-the-point book so I will spend enough time to give you a good foundation and then move on.

We'll evaluate different health practices within the context of stress. Why? Well here's the simple explanation:

Anything that increases stress ➜ Bad

Anything that decreases stress ➜ Good

So if the effects of accumulated stress (emotional, chemical, and/or physical) interfere with and break down the body's ability to function normally, then the first thing we want to do is *make sure we don't add any more.* So anytime you're considering doing *X* in order to get healthier, you need to pass that idea through the stress litmus test. If it will raise stress levels, don't do it!

How do you know if you're stressing yourself? Good question! Essentially, the symptoms of being under chronic stress mimic those of having a low metabolism.

Here is a brief list of things you can monitor (without obsessing about it!). The presence of these signs indicates things are going in the wrong direction:

Body temperature: Forget 98.6 degrees. Most people these days wish they could get that high. One of the ways you know your metabolism is decreasing is that your temperature will drop. Take your oral temperature first thing in the morning before drinking or brushing your teeth—98.0 and above is nice and a good sign that your engine is running at a nice clip. Upper 97s isn't horrible but signs you need work. Lower 97s into the 96s means you have the metabolism of a sleepy elephant seal. Establish a baseline and then as you make changes to your lifestyle, see how temps change in response.

Quality of sleep: When stress hormones are going gangbusters you'll tend to wake up in the middle of the night, usually in the 1:00 a.m. to 4:00 a.m. range. You might even have the experience of waking up at the exact same time. There was a stretch of time in my life when I would wake up nightly at exactly 3:15 a.m. I mean to the minute! It actually was freaking me out a little because I didn't understand how that was possible and that was the same time the dude from *The Amityville Horror* would wake up every night as he was losing his sanity. I eventually learned that adrenaline peaks during that time and I was stuck in a precise pattern. You know you are under some stress when you wake up routinely. You know you're *really* under stress when you wake up anxious and can't get back to sleep.

Feeling of warmth: Feeling cold (especially in the extremities) is another sign of stress and a slowed metabolism. If you frequently find yourself with cold hands and feet and are always layering up even in mild temperatures, your metabolism is likely low.

Other things to pay attention to as you assess your metabolic state are energy levels, motivation, presence of fatigue, dry skin, food hypersensitivities, constipation, and anxiety/depression.

Oral temperature is probably the best and easiest way to keep tabs since it gives you a number to compare. Remember though, if you start getting all OCD about your temps, you'll defeat the purpose.

So with that in mind, let's dive in.

Part II

....

DOWN THE RABBIT HOLE

Diet

When it comes to attempts at improving one's health, the diet is almost always the primary focus and is usually the gateway to other obsessive practices.

The trend over the last decade is hyperfocusing on diet when looking to assign blame and/or find cures for any health problems. Diet and nutrition has been a growing focus for decades (which is not necessarily bad) but in the last few years it's turned into an obsession. Food is everything. All things are caused and cured by food. In fact, some foods are assigned magical healing powers and some are even classified as "superfoods."

The problem is that everything you're eating is wrong. *Everything.*

Carbs? Nope, they cause diabetes, Alzheimer's, cancer, heart disease, and obesity.

Grains? Nope, they cause depression, insulin resistance, inflammation, and autoimmune disorders.

Protein? Nope, that causes cancer and diabetes.

Fat? Nope, polyunsaturated fat causes inflammation

and animal fats are unhealthy because the animals were grain fed.

Fiber? Nope, damages gut flora and interferes with mineral absorption.

Vegetables? Nope, vegetarianism has not been demonstrated to have any advantage and often results in nutritional deficiencies.

Fruit? Nope, fructose will kill you, don't cha know.

Nuts? Nope, high in phytic acid, which impedes mineral absorption.

Beans? Nope, they also have phytic acid, and since they're carbs, will give you the diabeetus.

Sugar? Nope, haven't you heard that sugar is addictive and is the root of all the world's problems?

Cheese? Nope, too much saturated fat and cholesterol and causes heart disease.

Butter? Nope, high in fat and causes heart disease.

Milk? Nope, promotes inflammation and is high in fat.

And let's not forget these other life and death considerations beyond simply what category of food we're eating.

We should also avoid at all costs: gluten, yeast, GMO products, artificial sweeteners, preservatives, additives, dyes, trans fats, high fructose corn syrup, salt, nitrites, nitrates, and acid-forming foods.

Not only do we need to focus on what we eat and what we need to avoid, but we also must consider how much we eat and how often. Don't eat too much, don't eat too little, don't eat too often, don't eat too infrequently.

Think you're done? Oh no. We also have to consider where the food comes from and how it was processed.

For animal foods we must know: Was it free-range? Grain fed? Grass fed? Pasture fed? Seed fed? Fed antibiotics? Given hormones? Outdoor bred? Raised in a pen? How big was the pen? Were they separated from the mother? Were they happy? Is it organic? How were they processed? By machine? By hand? At a factory? At a farm? Is it sustainable? Was it line caught? Net caught? Did any dolphins get caught in the net? Did any people get caught in the net?

For anything that grows we have to know: Is it organic? Were there pesticides used? Herbicides? GMOs? Did they use Monsanto seeds? Was it fair trade? Did it come from a supermarket? A farm market? Were there folk singers at the farm market? What fertilizer did they use? Was it handpicked? Was it hand-picked with love?

So what it comes down to is this—*anything* you choose to eat is bad for you and will likely result in disease. In fact, depending on what you read, *everything* has been linked to cancer, diabetes, inflammation, obesity, and cardiovascular disease. No matter what type of food you eat, how much you eat, how often you eat, or what you avoid, you are making a grave mistake. Have a nice day.

After years of exhaustive study and taking all the experts into account, I thought I had come up with the list of foods that everyone agreed were healthy. In fact, I was prepared to write a diet book including recipes to help all those searching for the holy grail of optimum health and those looking to finally shed that stubborn fat and achieve their God-given destiny for hotness. I was going to title the book *The List* and it would have sold a gazillion copies.

Admit it—you want to see the list, don't you?

Alright I'll show you but please realize this list has

been proven invalid so don't follow it!

The list of foods all diet gurus agree is healthy:

» Kale

» Grapefruit

There you go.

But again, just before publication of *The List,* and before production of the follow-up books, *Living the List*, *The List Dessert Book*, and *The List Lifestyle: What to Do When No One Will Talk to You Anymore Because You're Psycho and Your Breath Smells like Ketones* was to begin, I stumbled upon an article in the magazine *Women's World* while standing in line at the Piggly Wiggly: "Is Eating Too Much Kale Poisonous?" by K. Aleisha Fetters.

The first two paragraphs were all I needed to read:

> Right when you thought kale was the most perfect food known to (wo)man, a story comes along that says, "No, actually, it could poison you."

> The Mother Jones story, titled, "Sorry, Foodies: We're About to Ruin Kale" is going gangbusters. In two days, it's already rounded up more than 35,000 Facebook shares and is taking over Twitter,

suggesting that kale consumption commonly leads to too-high levels of thallium, a toxic metal, in the blood—and that that leads to chronic fatigue, skin problems, arrhythmias, gluten sensitivity, and Lyme disease. Yikes.

So obviously my integrity would not allow me to proceed with *The List* line of books and products. I mean, I could have *killed* somebody!

A short time later I happened upon this article in the peer-reviewed and prestigious journal *Women's Health* while in line at 7-Eleven:

"The Fruit That Can Kill You" by Alexandra Duron

Filling up on grapefruit might help you drop a few pounds, but proceed with caution: It could be hazardous to your health. Turns out, eating grapefruit can cause serious—even life-threatening—side effects if you mix it with any of 43 drugs, according to a new study published in the *Canadian Medical Association Journal.*

Imagine my chagrin when I learned that there was now *not a single food in the entire world* that all the experts could agree was good for me.

The problem is that members of the public at-large are basing their lifestyles on stuff that other people just make up. No really. Here's how it works:

Somebody comes up with a theory → they put it out there for public consumption → other people read it and say, "That sounds good" → they repeat it → more and more people read it and say, "That sounds good" → they tell two friends, and so on, and so on → theory now accepted as fact.

That's basically it.

In the past it used to be more difficult to spread bad advice around because you'd have to write an entire 400-page book, get it published, and sell it in bookstores for $25 to pull it off. Today, however, with the rise of the Internet, nonsense can rock around the globe before you can say, "Munchausen."

I get that it can be very confusing. Look, I've been doing this my entire adult life so I'm a little better versed with this health stuff than most but even I get befuddled at times. Have you ever had the experience of reading a book or article espousing a diet theory, and then after finishing, think, "That's it! That sounded so right it has to be the answer!" only to read another book or article espousing the exact opposite opinion and think, "That's it! That sounded so right it has to be the answer!"? Yeah, me too. They can sound *so* convincing!

This is why people get so whipsawed trying to discover the truth about diet and health. No matter what wacky health regimen you investigate, there will be a collection of people who did great on it, and many more who failed. Read forums and comment sections of *any* health article and you'll routinely see something like the following: "Adding crushed pork rinds to my kimchi smoothies completely cleared up my acne!" followed by, "Adding crushed pork rinds to my kimchi smoothies gave me horrible acne!"

Pick a diet theory, any diet theory, and you can construct a convincing argument using assumptions, conjecture, cherry-picked sections of cherry-picked studies, a little truth, and some good ol'-fashioned bullsh*t.

The lesson in this? Take what you read from "experts," whether doctors, gurus, authors, trainers, or neighbors with a *bite-size grain of salt*. No one has cornered the market on diet truth and if they say or act like they have, you need to *head for zee hills*! Most diet theories (and that's what they are, theories) have some good points but they are all incomplete and *none* of them are right for everybody.

Eventually, though, one of these diet gurus will get to you and you'll want to give it a try if you haven't already, and what starts out as a desire to get healthier and lose some weight can quickly degenerate into a mess, which is what I mean by the term "rabbit hole." There are two main scenarios that can start you down the path of doom.

You try something and it turns out to cause additional problems. Not only do you have to figure out how to fix the original issues but now you've got additional problems to solve. Each new wrinkle you try, whether adding something in or taking something out of your diet, will simply increase the number of variables making the puzzle more complex, hence going down the rabbit hole. You can quickly find yourself in the same place so many are stuck these days, in metabolic quicksand where nothing you try seems to help and you just keep sinking. Not good.

You try something and it "works" so you let it ride. By works I mean you get a result you're happy with. You lose some weight. You get some energy. Your mood improves. You have less flatulence. Whatever the benefit, the natural tendency for many is to think, *What else can I do to become even better?!* The positive results and improved life experience of the first thing you tried motivates you to learn more about how you can hack this body and make it shine. You begin what I call the "quest for optimum," which in my experience is like trying to find the end of a rainbow. The preoccupation of diet and health morphs you into an obsessive bore driven by your list of self-imposed rules.

In fact, in the last few years this has become so prominent that there has even been a name given to this "condition." I love the description in Karin Kratina, PhD's article "Orthorexia Nervosa" from the National Eating Disorders website:

> Those who have an "unhealthy obsession" with otherwise healthy eating may be suffering from "orthorexia nervosa," a term which literally means "fixation on righteous eating." Orthorexia starts out as an innocent attempt to eat more healthfully, but orthorexics become fixated on food quality and purity. They become consumed with what and how much to eat, and how to deal with "slip-ups." An iron-clad will is needed to maintain this rigid

eating style. Every day is a chance to eat right, be "good," rise above others in dietary prowess, and self-punish if temptation wins (usually through stricter eating, fasts and exercise). Self-esteem becomes wrapped up in the purity of orthorexics' diet and they sometimes feel superior to others, especially in regard to food intake.

Eventually food choices become so restrictive, in both variety and calories, that health suffers—an ironic twist for a person so completely dedicated to healthy eating. Eventually, the obsession with healthy eating can crowd out other activities . . . and become physically dangerous.

Ouch. Don't know about you but I've certainly been there and done that (more on that later). Do you see yourself in that description? C'mon, don't leave me hanging. If that description hit a little close to home, that's okay. There's hope for you yet!

Could it be that our obsession with diet has accomplished nothing but given rise to a society-wide eating disorder?

I believe that we have become so obsessed with "all things food" for several reasons:

It's easy for "experts" to sell. There's not a lot of money to be made by telling you to go home and work on your stress. A new diet theory though? *Cha-ching!* That's easy pickins.

People accept it. We love to blame outside factors for our shortcomings. We're an outside-in kinda people. We don't want to look inside and self-examine. We'd rather blame food.

It gives us a sense of control. I can track my diet meticulously. Calories, protein, carbs, fat, and fiber are *all* present and accounted for. I might be living with relentless psychological, emotional, and spiritual pain, and trauma, but I'm going to bury that and just obsess about my how many grams of polyunsaturated fat I ate for lunch today. Much like people with anorexia that starve themselves, it's really not about the food. It's about gaining a sense of control over one's life.

It distracts. Similar to gaining a sense of control, focusing on diet allows you to feel like you're taking steps to be healthy and improve without having to go *there*. The bad place. Inside. The fact is we *all* have baggage and issues and remember it's the accumulation of stress that is at the core of the problem. Until we go *there*, we'll just be spinning our wheels.

Another big difference between the diet focus of the past and the obsession we have now is that today all diet-related regimens are hardcore, painful, and downright masochistic.

Incorporate some vegetables in your menu? Increase the variety of foods to ensure consumption of a wider array of nutrients? Reduce intake of processed and lab-created substances and replace them with more natural ingredients? Nah, that's just not going to cut it.

» You need to consume nothing but pureed vegetables for thirty days followed by a "free day" where you get to eat an unsalted almond. Didn't you know you're a toxic, disgusting animal?

» You need to cut out *all grains*. You can never have bread again and your days of pizza, sandwiches, bagels, and cereal are *over*. Want some pizza? Make it out of ground-up cauliflower.

» Sugar is evil and you will never have it again. Did you know it stimulates the same part of the brain as heroin and cocaine and it's even more addictive?

> » You need to give up that morning cup of coffee you enjoy so much and sip cold gazpacho instead. It's better for you.

In other words, to be healthy you must completely obliterate any and all enjoyment from your food experience. Even though you're biologically driven to seek food, and eating is a major component of being a social animal, you are to deny all of that and embrace the discomfort of fighting your own biology. It needs to be next to impossible for you to go out for a meal. You'll know you've won when you eat all of your meals at home by yourself. You may be miserable but darn it you'll be healthy.

Hey, if you want health bad enough you need to *suffer* for it!

To paraphrase Irwin M. Fletcher, you don't need to be Sherlock Holmes to see that there is some serious psychological gymnastics at play here. Larry Holmes could figure it out. It's self-abuse all in the name of self-improvement. Larry Holmes would also know that abusing oneself is *not* the path to health.

The Hall Monitor

It's important to understand that the human body (as well as the body of any living organism for that matter) has what is called an innate intelligence that controls internal function, which is just a fancy term to describe the force inside that runs the show. It's life.

When you cut yourself, what happens? It heals. How did you heal? You probably have no idea but your body knows. What makes your heart beat? Your lungs breathe? What makes the immune system function and digestion happen? Innate intelligence. If you get the flu, what happens a few days later? You get better. How? The innate intelligence of the body.

Now you might say, "Hey wait, I thought the brain and nervous system controlled the function of the body," and you would be correct! I would just clarify that the innate intelligence (or "innate" for short) is what really runs the body and expresses itself *through* the nervous system. A dead body has a nervous system. What it doesn't have is life.

So when we're discussing the function of the body we have to keep in mind that innate is on the job and its purpose is to keep you going, regardless of how you feel about it. And unlike us, it knows what it's doing.

For instance, let's say you went to the gas station to fill up your tank and all of a sudden you get a cannot-be-denied hankerin' for some sushi. You look inside the mini-mart and lo and behold, right next to the shrink-wrapped subs and Hot Pockets you find a tray of California rolls. Sure the expiration date is today but hey, they usually build a couple of days' worth of buffer in there anyway, right?

Four hours later the first cramp hits the colon and the party is on. Both ends. Fast and furious.

So the questions you contemplate as you sit staple-gunned to the toilet are – are you sick or are you well?

From a functional standpoint, you're working perfectly. You ate gas station sushi and the critters on the sushi threatened to take you out. Your body determined that it was best for your survival that you ask those critters to leave *now* and it took measures into its own hands. It didn't care how you felt about it. It didn't care that you were on an airplane and there was a line at the bathroom. You might "feel" sick but you're actually functioning quite well.

This applies to our discussion about stress because your body, not you, gets to decide if what is happening is a stress event. You may be all excited about doing your new wheatgrass yogurt detox but it's innate that determines what your body does with it.

I have found the analogy of a hall monitor to be effective in helping people appreciate what goes on inside the body. The hall monitor is the innate intelligence of the body. The monitor roams your insides, vigilantly patrolling for any potential threats. Some of these threats include foreign invaders (i.e., your gas station sushi critters), changes in the environment, external threats, or psychological threats. Your body assesses the external threats using your senses and thoughts. This is why *how* and *what* we think play a *huge* role in whether we are in a state of stress.

So let's review.

The innate intelligence of the body is responsible for regulating all functions, including healing. Innate "flows" over the nervous system, which is why the nervous system is considered the master system of the body. Innate is constantly monitoring the body *and* the external environment (via the sensory nerves and organs) for any signs of threat. If innate (the hall monitor) senses a threat it will trigger a stress response. A little stress is no big deal (we need some air in the tire) but chronic, unrelenting stress accumulates, resulting in physiological changes that eventually lead to dysfunction and symptoms (the tire is overinflated).

So where we go from here is simple. If you want to make changes to improve your health, you need to do it in a way that does not alert the hall monitor! If the hall monitor catches on to what you're trying to do, it will spring into action and begin to resist.

If you've ever attempted to lose weight, then you've experienced this phenomenon. We'll cover weight loss more in depth a little later but the gist of it is that as soon as you cut calories, the hall monitor catches on and down regulates your metabolism to counter your effort because cutting calories is perceived as a threat. This is why you may lose some weight initially but soon hit a plateau. The plateau is the hall monitor resisting you. I know it's frustrating, but remember innate has a different priority than you. Although you want to look good at your reunion, your body wants to keep you alive.

What's even more frustrating is that many of the body's tricks and methods are unknown. We may have figured out a couple of things but we may not know much at all. The human body is quite complex and in many ways a total mystery, so since we don't have the knowledge to hack the system, we have to figure out how to get the result without tipping off the hall monitor. That means the only hope of losing weight is to do it *without* initiating a stress response.

Hopefully this is starting to come into focus. When you appreciate how incredibly sensitive the body is to changes and threats, is it any wonder that the health and diet regimens of today are driving people into a metabolic nightmare? I would go so far as to suggest that many times the stress caused by the "cure" is worse than the stress that caused the original condition. More often than not people would have been better off doing *nothing* as opposed to implementing some of these newfangled health ideas.

So let's look at some of the most common practices of the new school of masochism otherwise known as the pursuit of health.

Restriction of calories

The first diet mistake people make is to cut calories. Whether the reduction is intentional or not makes no difference. Even if the intent is not necessarily calorie restriction but rather to just clean up the diet the net effect will be fewer calories consumed. This is primarily because natural, and usually less palatable, foods have fewer calories coupled with the fact that they are less desirable so the drive to consume them is weaker.

For instance, if someone wanted to skip the usual four pieces of pepperoni pizza for dinner and instead have a baked potato with a little butter, they would have to eat five of them to equal the calories. Trust me—no one is sitting down to five baked potatoes. So even when calorie reduction isn't the primary goal, switching to an "eating clean" lifestyle will cut calories.

The hall monitor sees this coming a mile away and reducing calorie intake is one of the surest ways to trigger a stress response by the body.

When the stress response is triggered, your body will increase levels of certain hormones called, you guessed it, stress hormones—the primary chemicals released being glucocorticoids (cortisol) and catecholamines (adrenaline).

There are others involved but we're just going to focus

on these two. Both of these hormones are secreted by the adrenal glands. Since the body perceives a reduction of calories it responds by down-regulating your metabolism—your revolutions per minute (rpm) values at rest—accordingly, to hoard energy and keep you from starving.

One of the ways it does this is by dialing down the thyroid. The thyroid gland produces thyroid hormones and those are what dictate your metabolic rate. When the metabolic rate is high, you burn more fuel and energy. When the metabolic rate is low, you burn less fuel and energy. Pretty simple.

So if your body is in a panic because it thinks you're starving, what do you think it will do, raise your metabolic rate or lower it? Exactly, it lowers your rpm values until you're burning less energy to match the appropriate level of fuel intake. Pretty ingenious, actually.

If stress hormones go up, thyroid goes down. They pretty much act as opposites.

With this in mind, is it any wonder that with stress levels so high in so many people that hypothyroidism rates are skyrocketing? Any kind of stress will cause cortisol and adrenaline to rise, which acts to shut down the thyroid but if that weren't bad enough, when people start to diet and cut calories in order to "get healthy," they actually make it worse by adding even more stress, raising cortisol and adrenaline even more, and shutting down the thyroid even further. This is just one example of how attempting to do the right thing (clean up the diet or lose some weight) can backfire and make your health even worse.

This phenomenon is also why it is next to impossible to lose weight. We'll talk about weight loss a bit later, but the body's reaction to fewer calories by dialing down your metabolism is why you hit the dreaded weight loss plateaus. This is also why those that do manage to lose weight rarely keep it off. Your body will slow your metabolism to a crawl to resist starving and as soon as you relax your diet and start to eat normally again, the weight comes storming back due to the lower metabolic rate.

This lose weight/gain it back, lose weight/gain it back cycle is called yo-yo dieting and with each yo of the yo-yo, yo' metabolism gets a little bit slower. The lower your metabolism the fewer calories you need to consume per day. If you yo-yo diet long enough, you'll eventually get to the point where you gain weight no matter what you eat. Sound familiar? It's a bad place to be.

And if getting fat isn't enough low metabolism fun, here is a list of other symptoms of low thyroid/low metabolism for you to enjoy:

- » Fatigue
- » Lack of motivation
- » Dry skin
- » Mood disorders
- » Sleep disturbances
- » Lack of libido
- » Weight gain (even when eating "healthy")
- » Feeling cold (especially hands and feet)
- » Constipation
- » Changes in menstrual cycle
- » Infertility
- » Memory problems
- » Low body temperature

And I hate to tell you but this list is *short*. There are some sources that list *hundreds* of hypothyroid symptoms!

Oh, and one more thing just to add to the good times, there's a condition called cognitive dietary restraint, which is when cortisol is increased (stress response) simply from persistent *thoughts* of dieting and calorie restriction. So even if you never actually restrict calories, you can still experience the stress response just from thinking about it. Isn't that wonderful?

So what other kind of trouble can we get into?

Carbohydrate restriction

Aside from the reduction of daily calories that will likely occur on a low-carb diet (which will trigger a stress response), the fact that carbohydrates are restricted is, in and of itself, a stress trigger. Yes, this means cutting carbs will alert the hall monitor and cause a release of stress hormones.

Let's discuss some more fallout from living in this chronically stressed-out state.

Prolonged stress will start to interfere with normal function and result in symptoms and dysfunction. Remember, some of these symptoms will be present simply because of the accumulated stress of living (group 1), and some will be present because of consequences from adopting destructive health practices (group 2 if it was an innocent attempt at fixing health issues, and group 2b, or toobies, if it was all due to dieting and chasing the optimum health unicorn).

Other problems with living in a chronically stressed-out state, besides the fun of low thyroid function, are all too common food hypersensitivities.

Poor gluten. If gluten had feelings, I'd want to give it a hug. The little wheat protein gets blamed for everything these days. Inflammation, autoimmune disease, digestive disorders, killing Kennedy. In fact, an entirely new form of medicine has emerged called "Functional Medicine" where they charge you $5,000 to tell you to get off gluten.

Gluten is the go-to villain for most anyone having any kind of stress-related health issues. Now let me state clearly that it is possible to develop a legitimate gluten sensitivity. But let me state this even clearly, it's not the gluten—it's *you*.

I've known several people that indeed developed a not-so-subtle gluten sensitivity. In fact, if these people were to ingest gluten you could start the countdown before they would be sprinting to the bathroom with intense intestinal distress that would render it uninhabitable (the bathroom that is). It was undeniable. It's also fact that *all* of these same people were eventually able to return to eating gluten with no issues whatsoever. So while food sensitivities can and do happen, I don't believe it's because the food changed but rather the person eating it changed.

Any time I hear that humans were never intended to eat grains, I can't help but picture the famous painting of the last supper when the disciples ate bread and drank wine with Jesus. I guess if we were there, we would have seen some of them doubled over with intestinal cramps and a line to the bathroom (come to think of it, where *did* they poop in biblical times?). I can't believe Jesus had them eat something *so* destructive to the human body! And even worse, didn't he multiply five loaves of bread and two fish and feed 5,000 people as well? You mean to tell me that 5,000 people were hanging out eating fish sandwiches and everyone lived to tell about it? Maybe *that* was the true miracle!

If you are legitimately reacting to a certain food, then sometimes it's necessary to stay away from it for a while. I'm not suggesting you ignore the fact that you immediately crap your pants every time you eat a bagel and just keep eating them. Sometimes it's necessary to stay away from a certain food for a time to give your body a chance to reset. If chronic stress causes you to develop a food intolerance it *does not* mean that (a) you have to give up that food forever and (b) it's not safe for human consumption just because you can't handle it. Cutting it out of your diet for a few weeks might be all it takes. The people I have known with legit, bathroom-wrecking gluten sensitivities were *all* able to successfully go back to it after a few months.

By the way, one of the best ways to *create* a food intolerance is by cutting it out of your diet for a prolonged period of time so be careful what you restrict when starting your next diet.

Understand that food sensitivities can include potentially any food or food group. It's not just gluten. Gluten however is the cause celebre of the moment probably because of the anti-carb obsession that is raging in our society. Trust me, give it some time and everyone will move on to another villain.

Sensitivities are most likely another result of chronic stress.

Stress ➔ increased cortisol/adrenaline ➔ increased cytokines ➔ inflammation ➔ "spazzed-out" immune system.

Cytokines are pro-inflammatory chemicals released when stress hormones are present. Chronic elevation of these chemicals is associated with abnormal immune function including autoimmune conditions so when your immune system is in stressed-out, slash-and-burn mode it's possible to start reacting to things that pose you no harm.

Again, sometimes it's necessary to stay away from something for a short time but you want to re-introduce it as soon as you can. You don't want to go down the road of restricting too many foods because you'll paint yourself into a corner by inadvertently narrowing your available dietary choices to nothing but quinoa and flax seeds and that's no way to live.

Besides, even if you did develop a gluten sensitivity (which would surely be accompanied by other stress-related issues) that caused signs and symptoms, and you removed gluten from your diet and the symptoms improved, what does that mean? Proclaiming that getting off gluten healed your symptoms is like saying eyeglasses healed your vision. Is it really healing? Or did you just find a way to work around your newly acquired health issue?

If I'm afraid of drowning I either have to forever avoid water, or learn to swim. One solves the problem and one is a work-around. Which do you think would be the preferred solution?

So far we've established that restricting calories and restricting macronutrients will result in a stress response—I talked about carbohydrate specifically but it also applies to protein and fat. The stress created from restricting macronutrients will lead to more stress hormones, which increases cytokines, which jacks up your immune system and can make it go "kill 'em all and let God sort 'em out" on you and start attacking everything from food to your own organs.

Here's a scenario I'm seeing with patients more and more:

Mary starts to have symptoms of chronic stress and low thyroid such as weight gain, anxiety/depression, sleep disturbances, digestive problems, being cold all the time, achy muscles and joints, and fatigue.

Mary reads a book that convinces her that

carbohydrates are the cause of her problems.

Mary starts a low-carb, gluten-free diet.

Mary feels fantastic! More energy, less inflammation, sleeping better, pain free, and even some weight loss to boot! She feels ten years younger.

Mary continues with good results for a time— maybe a month, maybe six months, maybe a year (during which time she tells everyone she knows the greatness of low-carb livin').

Mary hits the wall and starts to go downhill.

Mary doubles down and gets more restrictive, trying to recapture the magic.

Mary feels worse.

Mary eventually gives up on the low-carb diet, and rapid weight gain begins due to the lowered metabolism.

Mary is now fat and pissed.

This is the tricky thing about starting restrictive diet regimens. Initially some good results are observed that convinces the person they've finally found their answer.

Depending on the person, they may do well for weeks to months or even years until the worm turns and they come crashing down. When this downward slide begins, the tendency is to buckle down even harder. Maybe initially it was just bread and sugar. Then it's dairy. Then starchy vegetables. Then all grains. Each new restriction is one more step toward orthorexia and further metabolic shutdown. Not good.

I suspect what is happening is that restricting carbohydrates causes a serious increase in cortisol, which on the outset feels good because cortisol is a steroid. Steroids snuff out inflammation and all the symptoms that go with it. People generally feel pretty good on steroids. Eventually though, the cortisol declines either through the adrenals tapping out or some other unknown process. When the steroid levels drop, so do you. Inflammation comes roaring back and now you've got an even lower metabolic rate to boot, which means you will start gaining weight while eating the same amount of food. The weight gain usually freaks people out and they reduce calories even more, digging the metabolic hole deeper and deeper.

What are some other causes of dietary stress besides restricting macronutrients and calories?

Fasting, including intermittent fasting (IF)

IF has gained in popularity and is more common in low-carb circles. This is where eating times are limited to certain hours of the day thereby creating a length of time where no food is ingested. Examples are only eating between noon and 6:00 p.m. (thereby "fasting" from 6:00 p.m. until noon the next day) or picking days of the week where no food is eaten. Are there benefits to IF? Maybe. The bottom line, though, is it's a major stressor. I tend to think that IF is probably okay for otherwise healthy and fit individuals but if you show any signs of chronic stress, then I would avoid it. Again, when in a stressed, low metabolic, low thyroid state, you *do not* want to pile on more stress.

The other problem with fasting or IF is that it still involves living with a hyperfocus on food, which never ends well.

Over-hydration

Hydration is a topic where the previously discussed phenomenon of "somebody makes something up and it gets repeated until accepted as truth" comes into play. This is also an area where health obsession starts to rear its head.

For the entire course of history, human beings . . . *er*, scratch that . . . the entire animal kingdom *including* human beings somehow managed to figure out how to get water down their gullets in just the right amount. To this day, animals know exactly when to eat, drink, urinate, move their bowels, and procreate, and they manage to get all of that done *without* Internet health gurus.

Then the experts showed up and now there are entire books on the topic of drinking water.

Seriously, this is when we as a society need to take a step back and have a reality check.

Have we become so disconnected with the functions of our body that we can't even manage to figure out we need to take a drink when we're thirsty? Do we really need authority figures who are just repeating what they read on the Internet to tell us when and how much to drink?

Here's my revolutionary new program for making sure you hydrate properly:

If you're thirsty, drink.

If you're not thirsty, don't drink.

Bam! There it is.

"Yeah but, Dr. P, you don't understand. I've read that once you experience thirst it's too late! And sometimes when you think you're hungry it's really dehydration and that we should drink half our body weight in ounces, which is unfortunate because I'm 300 pounds due to twenty years of yo-yo dieting, which means I have to drink 150 ounces of water a day, which is like, way over a gallon and they say coffee, tea, and soda don't count so when you add that in, I'm drinking so much I spend half the day in the bathroom and on top of it, I was told to eat nothing but vegetables, which are like, *all water* so now I'm probably up to two gallons a day, which means I have to carry a one gallon milk jug full of water around like a lunatic and now all I do is pee and crave salt and my body temperature is like two degrees above a corpse—do you have any pretzels? I need some pretzels! Wait, I have to pee!"

Yeah, we are *way* overthinking this thing.

If my "drink when you're thirsty, don't when you're not" program is just too simple for you, or if you're like, "You don't understand! I need rules. I need a system!"—then here's some more cutting-edge hydration knowledge for you—*pee is yellow.*

I know! I'm rockin' the body hacks!

When it comes to hydration it's important to realize that your body keeps a balance of electrolytes and fluid. This is why Gatorade was such a breakthrough back in the day. Gatorade was different because it added electrolytes (minerals) to replace those lost through sweating. When you drink too much fluid you effectively dilute the mineral concentration necessary for nerve and muscle function, so adding minerals to improve the performance of athletes was cutting-edge at the time.

Having overly diluted tissues is not good and will tank your metabolism. How do you know if your fluids are too diluted? A good rule of thumb is to check the color of your urine. Remember, pee is yellow. The saying is, "Don't eat yellow snow" not "Don't eat clear snow." I know you've had the rule of "keep drinking until you're peeing clear" rammed into your head for the last ten years, but again, it's just that it's been repeated so much, people assume it's true.

If your urine is clear, you either need to cut back on the fluids or eat more salt. If you have a nice yellow color, then you're just right. If it starts getting too yellow or even a brownish tint, then it's too concentrated and you need to drink some more. Also remember that some vitamins will give you fluorescent yellow urine, so don't mistake the presence of vitamin-induced highlighter-colored urine as the all-clear that you're good to go.

Really it's as simple as that. The fact that I have to spend time on this speaks to how ridiculous things have become. Drinking might be the most basic of animal functions yet we've completely lost trust in our intuitive biological cues to the point where we're so neurotically incapable we don't even know how to consume water anymore.

Later in the book, we'll discuss the concept of listening to our bodies to reconnect with biological signals so we can get back to functioning like capable, intelligently run organisms again.

Cleanses/detoxes

Cleanses and detoxes fit the current health narrative perfectly. I sometimes wonder if it's nothing but good ol'-fashioned self-loathing masquerading as self-care. I know professionals in the eating disorder recovery field are reporting that those with eating disorders should be very careful when experimenting with cleansing. Dr. Pauline Powers, who leads the scientific advisory committee for the Global Foundation for Eating Disorders, calls juice cleanses "the perfect pathway to disordered eating."

I've observed in the last few years that juicing, cleansing, and/or detoxing is being used by some people as a tool of punishment. A way to atone for one's dietary sins. A dietary spanking. Eat too much over the weekend? You must do a three-day juice fast. Consume some carbs or (*gasp!*) sugar at the birthday party yesterday? Your penance is a seven-day green shake detox.

"Bless me, trainer, for I have sinned. It's been one day since my last confession."

"One day?"

"Yes, well, I . . . this is hard . . . I . . . oh, I'm so ashamed."

"What is it, my child?"

"Yesterday, at lunch, I ate food that tasted good—and I enjoyed it. There were carbs and everything."

"I see," the trainer answers solemnly. "That *is* bad. Are you repentant?"

"I am! I am! I knew it was wrong and I am determined

to turn away from these sins. But it gets worse."

"Go on."

"When I weighed myself this morning I had gained 1.3 pounds."

A barely audible gasp is heard across the treadmill. "I see. Do a kale, cod liver oil wheatgrass spirulina superfood alkaline detox cleanse for the next two weeks followed by thrice daily coffee enemas and steel wool purification baths for another five days."

"Is that all it will take to purge the evil from my heart ... and colon?"

"It's a start. Go and sin no more."

Like everything else recommended by the health-osphere, cleanses and detoxes are Navy SEAL level bio-endurance tests. Have you noticed that *nothing* is ever easy? Apparently health can only be achieved through pain, difficulty, self-denial, and torture. Diet, exercise, cleanses, all of it. It's gotta hurt.

Health = masochism.

I believe this is intentional because it gives built-in cover for when these programs don't deliver results as promised. Anytime someone reports poor or no results it's always rationalized away because the person didn't do the program quite right.

"Oh you had an apple on day nine of your ten-day juice fast? No wonder you got poor results. All that sugar from the apple turned you acidic. If you would have just lasted one more day!"

Whether it's diet changes, cleanse protocols, or exercise programs, it always comes down to blaming the person if the results don't pan out.

Cleanses and detoxes are more quintessential examples of the "repeat it enough and it gets accepted as fact" phenomenon you see on the Internet. The idea that we're all nasty and toxic and that by doing these strange starvation protocols we will become clean and purified is really just a theory, and a disturbing one at that. People accept this because it plays into the self-loathing narrative. Not only are we fat, ugly, disgusting, lazy, gluttonous pigs but we're also filthy, toxic, and in desperate need of cleansing.

So looking at these from a stress point of view, would you think these cleanses and fasts *increase* or *decrease* stress? The gurus would have you believe they will decrease stress because you're "giving your digestive system a rest" and detoxifying. I would counter that there isn't a better example of how to throw yourself into a stress state then starving yourself, consuming massive amounts of fluids while at the same time ingesting zero salt. My goodness. No wonder people feel like they've been hit by a truck while doing these things (and no, it's not because you're detoxing).

I also believe that when you hear reports of people reaching euphoric states of well-being in the latter stages of a cleanse, that it's simply stress hormones spiking to high levels. Or heck, maybe it's an endorphin release as your body prepares you for death.

And for the record, I don't believe any of our organs need a rest. If anything needs a rest, it's our poor adrenal glands from having to work overtime trying to keep up with our "health" activities.

Let's sum up what we have so far.

If someone begins to suffer with the consequences of prolonged stress, it should be obvious that the best approach is to design a strategy that will begin to *lower* the stress levels and give the person an opportunity to heal. Makes sense, right?

Now think of the most popular advice plastered all over books, magazines, Internet, doctors' offices, and social media, which is to do the following:

» Lose weight

» Cut carbs

» Cut grains

» Cut sugar

» Drink a ton of water

» Lower salt intake

» Exercise

That is the current golden list for glorious health. Now let's put next to each recommendation whether it's a stress increasing or stress decreasing activity:

» Lose weight ➜ (stress increasing, metabolism lowering)

» Cut carbs ➜ (stress increasing, metabolism lowering)

» Cut sugar ➜ (stress increasing, metabolism lowering)

» Drink a ton of water ➜ (stress increasing, metabolism lowering)

» Lower salt intake ➜ (stress increasing, metabolism lowering)

» Exercise ➜ (stress increasing, metabolism lowering)

Do you see the problem? By the time you add all this "health" activity to your original problem you very well may find yourself in the metabolic quicksand up to your armpits. This is what I want to help you climb out of and hopefully prevent from ever happening again.

Look, our quest for optimum health (whatever that means) has led us down a dark and treacherous road. For many, the very act of eating has become a twisted, neurotic, and distressing experience that has to be replayed several times a day. Think back on your own life and picture how much time, energy, focus, and effort you have spent trying to get this part of life right only to fail time and time again. It's a no-win situation. We've awarded "expert" status to doctors, gurus, trainers, celebrities, and anyone else that claims to own the truth, and in turn they have juiced our brains of common sense and detoxed our critical thinking skills along with the supposed ten pounds of encrusted feces that line our dysfunctional colons.

Dieting is a stress. Thinking about dieting is a stress. Failing at dieting is a stress. Guilt and self-flagellation because you "can't stick with anything" is a stress.

Self-loathing is a stress. Using food to abuse yourself is a stress. It's all a big stress fiesta and you are the piñata.

Food is meant to be nourishment. Eating is supposed to be a stress-relieving activity. The simple act of digesting is enough to put you into an anti-stress, parasympathetic state (think of the nap/coma that follows Thanksgiving dinner). That's a good thing! But like many other aspects of life, we've totally screwed it up. I mean royally.

We'll get into suggestions for reversing this mess a little later but for now let me just suggest that you start chewing on this (pun intended):

> *You will never, ever, ever reclaim your health, your peace of mind, or your contentment until you eliminate the act of eating as a source of stress.*

Yes, that means stop dieting. Forever. Stop eliminating entire food groups. Stop eliminating macronutrients. Stop intentionally cutting calories. Stop obsessing about food. Stop setting up diet rules you must follow. Stop trying to find the *perfect* diet. Stop coming up with dietary villains. Stop trying to be "good." Just stop it all.

If you think about it, it's silly that we even have to be

discussing this.

Drink when you're thirsty. Sleep when you're tired. Move when you're energetic. Eat when you're hungry. Stop when you're full.

It's so anti-climactically simple yet beautifully elegant. There's no stress to be found in there anyway. Your dog even knows how to do it.

You should give it a try.

Weight Loss

Look, we need to have a serious talk.

I've got some news that you need to hear. At first you may not like what I'm about to say but if you can bring yourself to accept it you'll be well on your way to improving your health and life.

It's a paradox really. It doesn't sound like it should be true but it is. And if you can't or won't accept this truth then you will struggle for the rest of your life with self-esteem, disordered eating, stress issues, and your health in general.

Please let the following truth sink in.

It is virtually impossible—like, 97 percent impossible—to intentionally lose weight.

Now inhale deeply through the nose and exhale out the mouth.

Okay, I told you this would be hard at first. Hang in there, though, and hear me out.

Here are the facts from the research:

- » Of dieters who lose weight, 97 percent gain it all back and then some, after three years.
- » Exercise has been proven to be ineffective for weight loss.
- » Diets have been proven to be ineffective for weight loss (and actually make us fatter).
- » No one has figured out how to hack the human body to create lasting weight loss.

The science is convincing and the observations are indisputable. I'm sorry to report that lasting weight loss is an almost hopeless endeavor at this point.

Go ahead and take a few minutes if you must and have a good cry. I know. *There, there . . .*

Okay, now let's talk this out. As depressing as it may sound, there is a silver lining, a ray of hope. I said a moment ago that this is a paradox and the paradox is this—it appears the only hope for losing weight and keeping it off is if you can find a way to stop caring about it.

In other words, we're right back to the stress formula. The conclusions I have come to, based on the research, my own experience, and observation, is that any attempt to lose weight intentionally will simply throw your body into a stress response. Adrenaline and cortisol down regulate the thyroid, which slows down your metabolic rate, ultimately countering any attempt to create an energy deficit. The tease is that the early stages of a diet/exercise program will appear to work. Weight may come off. For a while. Ultimately, though, your body will get the last laugh. It will wait patiently for you to get done with your little health kick and then start marching back up the scale, obliterating your previous high and adding ten or twenty pounds to boot.

This scenario happens over 97 percent of the time. And the 3 percent that do maintain the weight loss do so at a heavy price—relentless daily exercise and constant strict dieting—living a neurotic lifestyle with food and weight being the number one focus of their lives, locked in a constant, daily battle against their biology. Doesn't that sound like fun?

If you find yourself in the common place where you are obsessed with losing weight and won't allow yourself to be happy unless you're a certain size, there's no other way to say it. You're in trouble.

The cold, hard facts are this—your weight is for the

most part determined by factors beyond your control. Genetics and heredity are the primary factors with stress levels and habits being secondary. Genetics are a done deal and how you were raised is water under the bridge at this point. So about all you can do is try and create an internal environment that decreases stress as much as possible so that maybe your body will, *on its own*, decide to drop some weight.

For the majority of people, spending a prolonged amount of time in a stressed state will lead to metabolic issues and weight gain. Aside from being anti-thyroid, cortisol stimulates the body to accumulate fat around the belly. It's about hoarding energy. As long as you're in a stressed state, the cycle continues. Again, it's a pile-on process for most of us. The stress of life accumulates, causing lowered metabolism and weight gain. We want to lose weight so we start dieting and exercising, which adds more stress. We ultimately fail, which causes more stress. We beat ourselves up and experience guilt (more stress). We try again to be "good" and lose weight (more stress). We fail again (more stress). And the cycle continues.

This literally goes on for years and/or decades for some. Stress on top of stress on top of stress. It's a no-win situation. The more you try, the fatter you become. This is why 97 percent gain it all back and then some. It's because you're fighting your biology and it's a fight you can't win.

It's really not as much about food as you might think. Overweight people don't necessarily eat more than thin people. It's primarily about genes, hormones, and metabolic rate. Sure you can have some outliers who are fat simply because they pound two dozen donuts for breakfast and wash it down with a container of chocolate sauce but that is by far the exception and not the rule (even though many of the public assumes all fat people are donut pounders). It's also not simply a matter of calories in, calories out either. This theory sounds like it should be true but it's simply not.

I'm a forty-six-year-old man and I have a six-year-old grandson (as of this writing). He weighs about forty-five pounds (all ribs and elbows) and I weigh 270. If you examined what we ate on a typical day you would find that our calorie intakes are not that far apart. You would expect that I out-eat him, and I do, but it's not by *that* much. Certainly not enough to be able to explain away with simple math.

I also find it curious why the men in a given prison,

who eat the same food in the same amounts (for the most part) for years can have wild fluctuations in body sizes. How can you have a bunch of skinny guys and at the same time have a bunch of big fat dudes if everyone's eating the same things? You can't blame the fat guys for hitting McDonald's and Pizza Hut every day, can you?

Most of the trite theories to explain fat people just don't hold up to scrutiny. The idea that all overweight people sit around drinking Pepsi and eating Pop-Tarts is nonsense and actually quite insulting. Oftentimes it's the overweight who are the most conscientious eaters in the room. I can also guarantee that one of the main reasons the overweight are the size they are is due to fallout from the countless attempts at losing weight.

And in case you think people are overweight out of laziness, studies have also demonstrated that exercise does not work for weight loss either. It's quite useless actually. I'm not saying exercise has no value because it surely does, but as a weight loss tool? It sucks.

Again, the only realistic hope you have of ever being a smaller size is to be a samurai warrior at reducing stress. By reducing stress hormones, you can increase thyroid function, increase the metabolic rate, live in a friendlier internal environment and then *maybe* your body will determine that you don't need to hold onto as much fat. If that happens, you'll find the scale going down all by itself. How long will it take? Who knows. Will it even happen at all? Don't know that either. That's for your innate to determine. All you can do is take steps to reverse the stress and try and raise your metabolic rate. We'll cover that in the last chapter.

Before you get too bummed out about the reality of weight loss, please understand just because you may be overweight or even obese that doesn't mean you are condemned to a life of sickness and disease.

When you look at the Centers for Disease Control reports for lowest mortality rates you'll notice that the lowest mortality rates are for those in the "overweight" and "obese" categories. Hmmm . . . also, while having a higher BMI has been linked to higher risk for type 2 diabetes, heart disease, and certain cancers, weight loss is *not* linked with lower levels of disease.

It's also interesting that the 2013 look AHEAD (Action for Health in Diabetes) study showed that people with type 2 diabetes who lost weight had just as many heart attacks, strokes, and deaths as those who didn't.

The moral of the story is that just because you are overweight doesn't mean you are going to suffer more disease than your thinner peers, and losing weight doesn't make all health problems go away. Heck, the mortality rates actually demonstrate that being overweight to mildly obese is *protective*. So if you're going to be stuck at a bigger size, at least don't lose sleep over the narrative that you're going to die an early death because the research doesn't support that conclusion.

Losing weight for most people really does come down to body image heavily influenced by a particular cultural preference. What people find attractive is subjective and arbitrary and it just so happens that in our culture we tend to take a "the smaller the better" approach to attractiveness. This is great if you happen to have drawn the genetic/hereditary cards that result in being small. It stinks if you drew the opposite cards. If you think about it, though, we could just as easily be a culture that finds chunky attractive and looks at thinness as undesirable. Then the thin people would have the eating disorders and the fat people could live their lives with a sense of contentment and unwarranted pride.

During the wee hours you would see a steady lineup of infomercials pushing products designed to get those poor, unhappy, unhealthy skinny people to change their lifestyles so that they too could achieve eternal hotness by gaining weight.

It's so simple, really.

If someone was genetically and hereditarily skinny we could solve the problem by just shaming them and telling them, "You know, you wouldn't look like that if you'd just eat more."

Or by blaming all of their health problems on their size, "Welp, Tammy's in the hospital again. She caught a cold and now she's got pneumonia, a collapsed lung, and a staph infection. *Tsk, tsk.* If only she'd get herself together and put on weight she'd be a lot heartier."

Or by threatening them with health stats, "You know, Larry, studies show that underweight people are much more likely to die than those of us who are overweight or even mildly obese."

Or by parading genetically or hereditarily overweight gurus on TV, Internet, and social media to instruct these defective, unmotivated beanpoles on how to gain weight and "take their lives back" by implying and/or declaring that the reason said guru looks so fat and hot is because of their awesome, dedicated lifestyle.

What you would see is the entire population of genetically skinny people turn into neurotic, food-obsessed, weight-obsessed maniacs. They would be chided by "experts" to "eat more, move less" and descend into depression when their attempts to eat more didn't result in permanent, dramatic weight gain.

"I ate as much as could but only gained five pounds this month! What's wrong with me?"

"You have to push through that plateau! Keep eating! Don't give up. Don't be a quitter! No pain, no gain! This isn't a diet! This is a lifestyle change!"

"But I'm not hungry! It's so hard to eat when you're stuffed full!"

"You obviously have a faulty biology and just need to overcome it. Maybe you need to do a cleanse?"

"What's that?"

"We're going to have you eat 8,000 calories a day of nothing but lard and butter for fourteen days."

"Won't that make me sick?"

"You may feel sick but that's just the detoxing."

"It sounds disgusting!"

"Don't worry, your taste buds will change. Remember, nothing tastes as bad as being skinny feels."

"But won't I start losing weight again as soon as I go back to eating normal?"

"Well, uh . . . you see . . . um, that's why you're going to switch to maintenance after you gain enough weight to make you hot."

"What's maintenance?"

"That's where you obsessively focus on your food and eat in a way that fights your biological drives until the day you die."

"That sounds like an awful way to live."

"You want to be healthy and attractive, don't you?"

"Uh, I guess so."

"Okay, then."

Do you see that how ridiculous it would be to think

that we could shame and horsewhip a genetically underweight person into becoming morbidly obese? Think of the thinnest, scrawniest person you know. Do you think you could come up with a plan to successfully *make* that person gain 100 pounds? How about 200? Yeah, me neither.

So if it's a ridiculous scenario to expect a genetically scrawny person to be able to gain 100 to 200 pounds, *why is it not just as ridiculous to expect the opposite?*

Let's not stop there, though! Let's put these poor people on national TV and, in front of millions, watch them stuff food into their mouths until they cry for mercy or, better yet, vomit. We'll weigh them at the end of the show and when they break down and cry because they ate so much they blew out their colons, but only gained two pounds we'll shake our heads somberly and whisper, "Too bad, she just didn't want it enough."

Not only will we pack 100 to 200 pounds on these people but we'll do it in just six months! We'll have some intense, genetically gifted, motivational fat trainers stand behind them as they eat, and cheer and berate them as they "change their lives." We can call it *The Biggest Sadist* and whoever gains the most weight wins the tiara and sash and will bask in the glorious confetti shower of awesomeness. The season will end after the finale and we'll be sure to *never* provide updates on the winners because the inconvenient truth is that they'll have re-lost all the weight by the time the new season starts. Losers. No willpower.

The unfortunate obsession our culture has with this virtually unwinnable fight generated $64 billion, that's *buh buh BILLION* in 2014 for the weight loss industry. I guess that's 64 billion reasons to keep you obsessed and flailing away. All that money spent and what do we have to show for it? Everyone's still overweight (probably more so), metabolisms are worse, stress is worse, and wallets are worse.

I don't expect that people are suddenly going to wake up and realize that the weight loss unicorn is imaginary and virtually unattainable and swear off diets forevermore. There are powerful cultural biases in play that will make it very challenging to give up obsessing about weight for those who struggle with weight issues. Like I said before, the only real hope you have of lowering weight and body fat levels is to make subtle changes that act to de-stress the body. The first of these de-stressing changes, ironically, is to stop obsessing about your weight!

Focus on health first and let the weight take care of itself. That may mean you end up losing some fat and inches over the weeks, months, and years, or it may mean no change at all. You need to make peace with that reality.

I realize that preaching this message is not going to generate $64 billion next year, which is why very few will echo my message.

Someone needs to level with you, though.

It may as well be me.

Exercise

Exercise is a good example of why *some* stress can be a good thing. If you remember from the bike tire analogy, you need a certain level of air pressure for the tire to function. If you have *no* air in the tire, then it's flat and useless. It's the same way with you and stress. The goal in life is not to eliminate *all* stress because then you'd be a lifeless lump. Stress can either get us *out* of bed or land us *in* bed, depending on the amount.

It also depends on how you feel about the stress that determines the effect it has on the body.

At work, the stress of a challenge you enjoy could be a good stress, while facing the wrath of a boss when missing an unreasonable deadline would be a bad stress. Seeing the suffering in the world could be a bad stress because it saddens you, or it could become a good stress if it stirs in you a sense of purpose.

It's all perspective. Your body doesn't know the difference between good and bad emotional and psychological stress. When something occurs in your life, your nervous system waits for you to assign a meaning to it before it determines what response to run. This is why attitude and your view of reality can make all the difference in the world as to how stressed your body becomes.

Exercise is no different, to a point.

What I mean is that the physical stress of exercise will take on different meaning to your nervous system depending on how you feel about it. For instance, if you reluctantly decided to start exercising out of guilt from your family, then it will likely be something you feel like you *have* to do as opposed to something you *want* to do. In general, if we do something we have to do but don't want to do, we won't enjoy it and probably won't stick with it very long. The effect that exercise has is largely determined by your attitude going in. It's no different than your job, your family, your friends, or any other aspect of life. If you enjoy something, the stress effect will be different than if you don't.

If you go to a job you dislike but feel as if you have to do it ➜ bad.

If you go to a job you love because you freely choose to ➜ good.

A planned visit if you can't stand your relatives ➜ bad.

A planned visit if you enjoy visiting and interacting with relatives ➜ good.

And likewise with exercise, if you go because you genuinely want to and enjoy the experience, then that will have a different effect on the body than if you dread the experience and have to drag yourself there through willpower and guilt.

For instance, a 100-yard sprint because you're scoring the winning touchdown in the Super Bowl versus a 100-yard sprint because you're running through the woods from a hockey mask-wearing Jason and his machete would produce two very different stress reactions. Technically it's the same physical activity—a 100-yard sprint. The only difference is how you feel about it.

Bringing it back to the real world—if you take a two-mile walk down a trail through the foothills near your home on a sunny 75-degree day, it would be a different stress experience than walking the same two miles on a treadmill staring at the sweaty back of the dude on the treadmill in front of you. So how you feel about what you're doing for "exercise" will largely determine the effect it has on you.

When it comes to physical activity, you need to choose activities that you genuinely enjoy because (a) you're much more likely to stick with them and (b) the stress effect will work *with* you and not *against* you.

While emotional and psychological stress is almost completely determined by how you feel and the meanings you attach to circumstances, physical stress can be a mixed bag.

The actual act of exercise is a physical stress and, just like any stress, there's good and there's bad. Let's set aside the aspect of how you feel about it for a moment and just consider the physical act itself. There's a fine line between physical activity being a building-up activity (anabolic) or a tearing-down activity (catabolic). Two major determinates for this are *amount* and *intensity*.

Remember, my goal is to give you a practical, concept-driven understanding, and not try and turn you into exercise physiologists. There have been volumes researched and published on this topic, so let's keep this reasonable and to the point.

The amount of physical activity is important because for exercise to be a benefit and build you up (increased muscle tissue, endurance, and strength), there needs to be appropriate rest so the body can recover from the stress of the exercise. How much activity and how much rest is completely determined by the innate intelligence of the body and encompasses a bunch of factors, many of which we don't even know. For instance, the age of the person, their fitness level, history of injury, genetics, current stress level, and historical stress levels.

As I'm writing this, it was just yesterday afternoon that I met a doctor friend of mine at my office. He texted me in the morning that he had locked up his lower back while working out the night before and that he was limpin' and hurtin'.

I met him at the office and he explained, "I wasn't doing anything out of the ordinary. Just in my basement lifting some weights like usual." He went on to add, "I think the problem was that I was behind on sleep this week and my nervous system couldn't handle the stress." Bingo.

So how much exercise is the right amount and how much rest is needed is a fluctuating amount depending on a lot of factors that must be assessed in real time. Sorry, you can't just listen to some doctor or trainer give blanket recommendations for *everyone* and assume that it's right for you.

So how are you supposed to know how much activity is the right amount and how much rest is needed? Again, it's a revolutionary yet little-known approach called "listen to your body." We'll cover this in more detail in the next chapter but for now let's just go back to the stress consideration.

Signs you need more rest and should back off the throttle:

Fatigue. While you should be tired and feel worked at the end of a workout, you shouldn't need to be carried to your car. You should also be able to snap back relatively quickly in the next day or two. If you're still tired days later, you overdid it and need more rest.

Excessive soreness. If your legs feel heavy, your knees ache for a week after your jog, and you can't reach around to wipe yourself due to muscle soreness, you overdid it. Back it off.

Lack of motivation. If you find you are having to give a Knute Rockne motivational speech to yourself simply to hit "play" on the DVD workout program, that's a neon-red flag that you're in a bad stress place. Your brain is begging you to stop.

Injuries. If you start having nagging injuries that never quite resolve, you need to dial it down.

No results. If you are working hard but find you see or feel no appreciable difference, you're overtrained. With appropriate stress-rest cycles you should get stronger, faster, and have increased endurance. If nothing changes, then you're tearing yourself down not building yourself up.

These are just a few clues that should be fairly self-explanatory. Again, we've had nonsense and goofy health practices marketed to us so hard and for so long that we've completely lost touch with the obvious.

Look, if you have *no* energy for exercise and the thought of going to the gym makes you want to take a nap, then there's a good chance you're in an overstressed state. If your body is in stressed-out survival mode, the *last* thing it wants is for you to squander what little reserves you have on high-intensity activities that produce nothing. Spend 500 calories hunting to prevent starvation? Have at it! Spend 500 calories on an elliptical machine so you can be hot someday? *Nuh uh.*

Intensity is not so much how *long* you perform an activity but how *hard* you perform that activity. Thirty minutes on a treadmill walking like your shoelaces are tied together is a different intensity than jacking the incline to max and cranking the speed up to ten. A balls-to-the-wall workout requires more rest and recuperative time than a mellow, less intense one, and is a much bigger stress to the body.

Again, some stress is good but too much is bad and everyone has their own personal line where a stress turns that corner. I know watching the infomercials for Insanity or P90X while you're slouched in a Barcalounger covered in Cheetos dust is inspiring but you need to think this through.

Unless you are already an athletic, highly fit individual, the likelihood of overtraining and creating a stress disaster for yourself is about 100 percent. If you are in an overstressed state, the *last* thing you want to do is perform high-intensity exercise for an hour a day. Are you kidding me? I can't tell you how many patients I see for exercise-induced injuries. And not the "I twisted my ankle playing basketball" type, either. Injuries as a direct result of performing complex activities at too high intensity for too long and without enough recovery time. All because they got swept up in the ridiculous idea that in order to improve their fitness and health they had to endure a "boot camp."

We're right back to the over-the-top, vomit-inducing torture sessions all in the name of "getting healthy."

It completes the trifecta of terror:

Masochistic, hardcore calorie and diet restrictions +

Masochistic cleansing and detoxing protocols +

Masochistic boot camp style, grind you into the ground with no rest exercise obsession

= Health

Okay, sure. Honestly, if *this* is where health comes from, I'm not sure I want it.

Knowing what you now know about stress, can you see why the above recommendations are head-scratchingly absurd?

Just like any stress, overtraining causes cortisol increase (as well as testosterone and progesterone decreases), which leads to all the usual fun that comes from being overstressed with a crashed metabolism. Add to that the likelihood of physical injury when overtrained and it becomes even more delightful.

One more point about exercise. Just like size and body fat-level tendencies, everyone has their genetic limits when it comes to physical abilities. Again, without getting too specific, understand the overall point I'm trying to make. Some people are able to do things that others can't.

For example, something I've noticed over my twenty years in practice is that there seems to be a magic line when it comes to jogging and running. Regardless of body size, level of fitness, or motivation, I've observed that a majority of joggers I see, some who have been running their entire lives, start having problems when running farther than a 5K (3.2 miles). Keep the distance under a 5K and all is quiet and right with the world. Go over a 5K and the aches, pains, and injuries start showing up.

Now for those that dream of running a marathon this is frustrating because the pain and injuries stop them from progressing to their goal, but the fact is that going past three or four miles causes a breakdown in their structure and function. It just does. Then there are those that seemingly perform absurd feats of strength and endurance with nary a sore muscle.

I remember several years ago going to a specialty running shoe store outside of Cleveland, Ohio. The salesman, a twenty-something year old, casually stated in the course of conversation that he ran 26 miles that morning before coming in for his eight-hour shift. I was stunned! If most human beings ran 26 miles they would at the *very least* be shot for the day. This guy just grabbed a shower, ate a sandwich, and sauntered on in for work!

So there *are* exceptions out there that can handle extreme levels of physical activity and hold up under the demand. Key word being *exceptions*. For most of us, however, there are limits. My point is this—be reasonable in your expectations. If you are regularly experiencing pain and injury when crossing a certain level of activity, then accept it. There's nothing wrong with pushing the envelope now and then to see if you can reach new ground but don't be dopey about it.

I can't tell you how many patients I've had over the years

that, after giving up on their obsessive, self-imposed exercise demands, experienced a dramatic increase in health and well-being. It is common at this point to hear something to the effect of, "I stopped running five miles a day and switched to yoga and now I never get back pain anymore," or "I feel so much more energy since I stopped going to the gym every day."

Exercise is a stress. Activity is a *good* thing and necessary for health. The trick is to find that balance so that your physical activity builds you up and doesn't tear you down.

One more point (really this is the last one). Unless you are a professional athlete, training for the Olympics or somehow make your living being ultra fit, it is really a waste of energy to be obsessed with exercise. I get why players in the NFL need to train for hours a day. I get why Olympians need to make training their major focus. But you? Me?

Just like during our discussion of health in general, when is enough good enough? So you can run five miles. Then you need to run ten. Then a half marathon. Then a marathon. When does it end? I get why fitness is important but fitness should be a means to an end, not the main point of life. You exercise to live, not live to exercise. I see so many people crossing that line into obsession. Like constantly topping your last feat of strength somehow gets you bonus points.

It gets back to the whole narcissism thing. Be careful because what may start out as an innocent desire to increase strength and endurance can quickly descend into a weird place where you're scrutinizing yourself, admiring yourself, and otherwise thinking about yourself constantly and posting selfies forty-seven times a day. You may not see the dysfunction, but trust me, everyone else does.

So it comes down to this—what are we to do?

We've covered a lot about a lot and I've hopefully prepared you for the next chapter, which is where we'll discuss my suggestions to regain, keep, or protect your health going forward. If I've done my job well, my recommendations should be a little anticlimactic and obvious. In fact, I'll bet you can probably guess many of them. That's good. It means you're thinking with a clear head and not with one clouded by a swirling vortex of health guru drivel.

Part III

So What Do We Do Now?

The last ten years have seen an explosion in conditions related to stress overload. Interview enough people and the recurring themes of unexplained drops in thyroid function, food sensitivities, depression, anxiety, digestion problems, fatigue, weight gain, blood sugar abnormalities, aches and pains, pain syndromes, headaches, and chronic inflammation are unavoidable. It's almost becoming the norm.

One of the questions on my office intake form asks the new patients to rate their stress on a scale of 1 to 10, 10 being worst. The vast majority rate in the 7 to 10 range with an alarming number rating their stress level at a 9 or 10. This may seem incidental or just another notable finding on their history, yet it's anything but. In fact, it's probably the most important question I ask.

I don't know that anyone who knows anything about health would argue that stress is the ultimate cause of declining health. It doesn't get a lot of attention and doctors don't spend a lot of time on it because quite frankly, no one knows what to do about it. There are no nice, tidy little answers, and no pills for which to write a prescription. Therefore, we brush it aside, assigning it elephant-in-the-room status but look past it to pretend that other things are really the problem.

"If only people would stop eating sugar."

"If only people would exercise an hour a day."

"If only people would lose weight," the health authorities proclaim.

"If only they would stop eating eggs ... wait, I mean *start* eating eggs ... no, *stop* eating them, I mean, uh, *start* eating them but just the whites ..."

Meanwhile the naive public gets led around by the nose and their health declines, all the while blaming themselves for being defective, lazy, and uncommitted when their attempts at implementing this carnival of contradiction fails.

So what do you say we try something else?

I'm going to give you some recommendations on what I see as the most important things to do to give yourself the best chance of living a healthy life. I stated at the beginning of this book that my perspective comes from not only research, my twenty years of practice, observation, and common sense, but also from my own personal experience, which you might find interesting.

You see, virtually *everything* I rail against, *everything*

I poke fun at and ridicule, *everything* I blame for creating much of the health challenges we see today, *I've been guilty of myself.*

There I said it.

And not only have I been guilty of *doing* these things, but I've been guilty of recommending them to others as well. *Ouch.*

The dieting, low-carb, gluten-free, paleo, cleanses, detoxing, all of it. I've been there, done that, and got the mug, T-shirt, and wrecked metabolism to show for it. I guess that's why I feel I can make fun of this stuff. I earned the right!

In many ways I'm the typical toobie. No real health problems to overcome, but I wasn't happy with my dimensions. I've always been a big boy and tended to carry an extra twenty pounds of fat. Even though I was a runner, played sports, and lived an otherwise active life, the twenty were always there.

Because I'm a chiropractor and therefore a little more aware of "alternative" thinking when it comes to health, I toyed with the concepts of paleo, low-carb, gluten-free, and acid-alkaline several years before most people had even heard of those things. Don't get me wrong, I didn't invent those concepts but I was just aware of them before the mainstream caught on. I tried it all.

In fact, in 2007 I wrote a book entitled *The Year I Lost It*, which was the story of my attempt to lose one hundred pounds. I basically wrote a weekly e-mail update along my year-long effort so people could follow along on my attempt to experience the good, the bad, and the ugly of my journey. I was even featured on the Fox News station out of Cleveland. I had hundreds of people following my story. I was an inspiration to many! By the end of the year I had lost about eighty pounds and considered the journey a success.

Throughout the '90s, my wife Susan and I dealt with a lot of stress. One of the larger periods of stress was when our son Christopher went to Iraq. He was a marine and when the war started in 2003, he was there on the front line as the invasion began. I remember one Tuesday morning Susan received a static-filled phone call. It was Chris and he was calling from a satellite phone as he and the rest of the initial invading force were stacked at the Kuwait border awaiting orders to go in. He said he was calling because we wouldn't be hearing from him for a while and he wanted to say good-bye. As he was talking, he abruptly yelled into the phone, "I gotta go!" and hung up. Sue sat there in shock as we wondered what had happened. A few minutes later the phone rang again and it was Chris. "Sorry about that," he said, "a missile just flew over our heads and we had to get our gas masks on." He then said good-bye and hung up.

We then spent the next months obsessively watching the scroll on Fox News. They would publish the names of those killed in the invasion and we would sit there praying his name wouldn't show up. We also jumped every time the phone rang, looking at the caller ID, and sighing in relief when it wasn't a government phone number. So yeah, good times. That was also the time that Sue started having issues with her thyroid.

She was diagnosed with Graves' disease (an autoimmune disease causing hyperthyroid) a short time later and we spent the next few years trying anything and everything to get it reversed. Around 2008 she started having some acute digestive distress and after researching high and low we finally figured out it was a gluten reaction. No doubt about it. Any gluten and it was an instant trip to the bathroom.

We tried this "no-gluten" thing and lo and behold, it worked! No more digestive distress. Since so little was known at the time, Sue started a gluten-free support group in our town and a good number of people attended every month to discuss and receive support for this relatively new and unknown issue.

One of the more embarrassing moments was when Sue was at lunch with a close friend at the time. They sat down in a booth at Applebee's and ordered salads and when the server came to check on them, the friend asked the server if she was sure the salad dressing was gluten-free. The server didn't know what she was talking about so the friend asked to see the container the salad dressing came in. They both walked toward the kitchen (which was on the other side of the restaurant) and she waited by the kitchen entrance. The server came out with a big commercial jug full of dressing and the friend proceeded to read the label. She then looked up and yelled, "*Stop!*" while extending her arm, palm out. "*Don't eat the dressing! There's gluten in the dressing!*" Sue was mortified and wanted to crawl under the table as the entire restaurant, including the full bar, turned to look at which person this lunatic was yelling.

We even went on a couple of cruises while doing the no-gluten thing and had to call ahead to the cruise line and inform them of her dietary restriction. The cruise line graciously accommodated her and even arranged to make gluten-free bread to be served at our dinner every night. While very nice of them the bread tasted like a cereal box. So yeah, we understand that gluten issues can be real.

About nine months after going gluten-free, she decided to test it one day in a spontaneous oh-the-hell-with-it moment where she decided she wanted pizza with the rest of us. So she dove in. Minutes went by, then an hour, then several hours. No digestive problems. Could it be?

She had a bagel the next morning for breakfast. All was quiet. Long story short, it's been eight years and no more signs of gluten issues. (No, going gluten-free did not reverse the Graves' disease. We had her thyroid removed in 2009 and she's been fine ever since with a little help from Synthroid.)

So the foundation of our health concerns (her thyroid, my weight) was brought on by intense stress over a prolonged period of time. It seemed like the stressful challenges and crises were stacked one behind the other like a line of jets coming in for landing at a busy airport. As our symptoms progressed, much like the descriptions you read in this book, the more we tried to counter them. In 2009 after I had lost the eighty pounds, we experienced a whole new level of stress through some tragic family circumstances, and one year later I had gained back all the weight I had lost, plus an extra twenty pounds for my trouble. It was a combination of a slowed metabolism from losing the weight plus the added stress of the new crisis plus the fact that I was distracted and couldn't spend every waking moment obsessing about food and I didn't have the energy to spend on the self-discipline required to keep it up.

Through our attempts at solving her thyroid issue and me trying to lose weight, we tried just about everything we could think of including everything I've brought up in this book. I even had knee surgery in 2012 for a torn meniscus that happened, you guessed it, participating in an exercise boot camp.

So everything I talk about I've not only experienced firsthand but have watched countless patients struggle with as well. The recommendations I have for you, I have done myself. It's been a few years and I am still in the process of repairing the fallout from all of my attempts to get healthy. I hope you follow me.

A Stress-Centered View of Health

As I often tell my patients, "If you just assume that everything is stress, even if you're wrong now and then, you'll still be healthier and happier than anyone you know."

That suggestion is the same one I'm making to you. If you are considering making any changes to your routine (doesn't matter what area of life really) the question to ask is, "Will this change reduce my stress load or add to it?" If the answer is "add," then don't do it.

When I say add stress, I'm talking about the big picture. For instance, if you are considering changing jobs from one you can't stand and find boring to something stimulating that pays more, but at the same time find it stressful to change your routine, I'd say the bigger value wins. Sure you're adding some short-term stress by changing it up, but in the long run you will come out way ahead by having a job you love going to every day. So don't get bogged down with those kinds of questions. Don't overthink it.

Decreasing the stress load is like peeling an onion. It's a layer thing. When we start to tackle this job, we'll start with the outer layers of stress, which are the things we can easily stop or start. I suggest we begin with looking at your diet and exercise habits.

Let's agree that when making decisions about diet and exercise, we'll choose habits that honor the body. This means we're done with self-abuse and masochism in the name of health. The pursuit of health is not synonymous with torture. If you've let your health slip over the years you do *not* need to be punished before you're allowed to recover.

Choosing habits that honor the body means not doing things that overstress your system. Also keep in mind that you were probably overstressed before you tried to fix it, so our starting point is most likely pretty deep in the hole. Job one is to start climbing out of it.

We do this by doing the *opposite* of what got us here. Increased stress hormones tank our thyroid and metabolism. To get our thyroid and metabolism coming back to life we need to start with the following:

» Eat
» Sleep
» Rest
» Properly hydrate
» Exercise appropriately

Eat. There's no way around it, you must eat and eat plenty. You don't have to purposely gorge yourself but you need to eat enough so that the hall monitor doesn't suspect a calorie shortage. This will probably be more than you're used to, especially at first. In fact, you may even have to deal with some guilt and fear issues because you've been taught to have an unhealthy relationship with food. Thanks, gurus. Eat everything too. Don't you dare say, "I'm going to do it!" and then eat thirty pounds of broccoli. Forget the good food/bad food thing and just eat. Eat what sounds good. It's *all* allowed. Give yourself permission to eat whatever you want. Trust me, you won't go nuts and blow out your rectum. You might initially indulge in some taboo goodies you've missed but you'll get over that quickly. The only reason you dream about ice cream, pizza, and Ding Dongs is because you've made them off-limits. If you're allowed to eat anything you want, you'll be surprised how much less you think about food.

Remember, rules simply make you obsess about them. If you're allowed to have pizza anytime you want, without limit, you might have it once a week and not even think about it the other days. The minute I say you can't have gluten, grains, or carbs so no pizza is allowed, guess what you're going to become obsessed with?

So eat *whatever* you want and *however much* you want. Don't hold back. Eat until you're satisfied. If you allow yourself to eat whatever and however much you want, guess what goes out the window? Bingeing. That's what dieters and people with unhealthy relationships with food do. They try and try to "be good," which means self-denial and eventually they slip up. When they slip up they think, "Well, I blew it today so I might as well get my fill because I'm back on track tomorrow!" So they proceed to binge. They binge because they're thinking, "This is the last time I get to eat this."

Do you really think you'll eat an entire pizza if you know you're allowed to get some any time you want? You won't.

Ultimately we want to get to the point where we eat according to our biological cues. You know, like all the other animals on Earth. Got a hankerin' for something? It's probably because that's what your body needs. Craving something salty? I wonder why. Craving something sweet? Something fatty? Learn to start listening to your body instead of intellectually overriding it because of something you read on a Facebook post or on a blog.

Eat *whatever* you want, *whenever* you want, and *however much* you want. Eat when you're hungry, stop when you're full. It's really that simple.

Give it time, though. If you've been on a restricted diet with restricted calories for a long time it might take your body a little time to wake back up and get in gear. That's okay. If you get a little digestive distress the first day or two don't panic and say, "See! It's the grains! The carbs! I knew they were deadly!" Just stick with it and see if you can push through to the other side.

See if you can start feeling the stress go down. See if you start sleeping better and deeper with less waking up during the night. See if your mood starts improving. Observe your energy levels and motivation. Don't be surprised or dismayed if you gain a little weight. That's normal when you're going through the process of healing. You can also track your morning temps as you start eating normally again. You should start to see your temps increase as you increase metabolism.

If you decide at some point to improve the quality of food in your diet, that's okay. Just make sure you're not eliminating any food groups and make sure you're not cutting calories (which tends to happen when you start "eating clean"). If you are going to incorporate more vegetables and low calorie foods in your diet, then you'll need to eat more.

Remember, your goal is to decrease stress so you can start the healing process. It's like turning the *Titanic*. It takes time. Please don't make this all about weight. You can think about weight later. Besides, until you reverse the never-ending stress response you won't have a prayer of lasting weight loss anyway. The research is clear. You can't starve off weight and expect it to stay lost. Statistically speaking you have virtually no shot. It's only by creating an internal environment of low stress that your body may decide to drop some excess weight by raising your metabolic rate.

Ultimate goal: To live your life focused on important things and *not* obsessing about food. To return to intuitive eating where you use your own biological cues to make decisions—eat what sounds good at the time, eat when hungry, stop when full. To ditch eating rules and to eliminate stressful emotions surrounding food such as guilt and fear.

Sleep. Sleep is an essential component of rebuilding and maintaining your health. Short yourself of necessary sleep and you're guaranteed to trigger a stress response. How much sleep do you need? Again, relying on your biological cues would be great, but if you've been disconnected from your body for a long time you might not even know how to do that! The answer I'll give you is "as much as you can get"—even as much as ten hours a night. The more the better, because the more sleep you get, the more recovery you experience.

I know, I know, you're busy. We're all busy. I realize you're not a kid and may not have the luxury of sleeping until nine every morning. Do what you can. If your wake-up time is fixed due to a job or school, then tinker with bedtime. Go to bed earlier. Start winding down sooner. Get yourself some blackout curtains and make your bedroom as dark as possible. Stop watching TV before bed and disconnect from your devices earlier. Make it happen. The extra sleep will pay off!

If you have trouble with waking up during the night, it's probably because of spiking adrenaline. Sugar and salt can help so you can either keep some pretzels by your bed to eat if you wake up or make sure and have some salty carbs before bed.

Ultimate goal: To sleep eight to ten hours a night, soundly and uninterrupted.

Rest. By rest I mean getting any non-nighttime sleep or down time. In an overstressed state where the goal is to rebuild and restore your health, it should be obvious that rest is an important factor. If sleep is restorative, then rest isn't far behind. This means you may need to dial back on the schedule a bit. Do you fill every waking moment with activity or chores? Do you have trouble just lounging on the couch for a while? Can you chill out and read a book? Do you always have to be working, working, working? Not to get too deep here but sometimes people maintain an unnecessarily frantic pace to their lives because when they stop and sit still for a minute, it gets emotionally uncomfortable—like they can't be alone with their thoughts.

I give you permission to calm down, be less productive, and waste some time doing nothing. Steal a nap when you can. Read novels. Do jigsaw puzzles. Work crosswords. Find something to do to chill out, zone out, and relax. It's exactly what a stressed-out body and mind need.

Ultimate goal: To spend time every day doing nothing productive and enjoying it. Find time to relax and do something calming such as reading, napping, or working on puzzles.

Properly hydrate. We covered this earlier but let me reiterate a couple of points. Don't overthink this. Diluting your fluids is not good and that is what happens when you drink ridiculous amounts of water. The problem becomes worse when you combine this with purposely avoiding salt. Drink when you're thirsty. Stop when you're satisfied. Oh, and don't avoid salt. You also shouldn't be sprinting to the bathroom every fifteen minutes. If you are, it's likely that your body is trying to dump water to rebalance your electrolytes.

If you don't trust your instincts yet, then use the yellow rule, as in, pee is yellow. Your urine should be a nice yellow, so if it's clear, you're probably overhydrated, and if it's its dark yellow you're probably dehydrated. It really doesn't have to be any more complicated than that.

Ultimate goal: Rely on biological cues to tell you when to drink. Don't intellectualize it. Use urine color as a guide.

Exercise appropriately. Exercise is not supposed to be a form of torture. It's supposed to be a controlled stress that stimulates your body to repair and become stronger. The repair happens during rest. If you don't get enough rest and repair time, then all you're doing is continuously stressing the body and you won't get any benefit. In fact, exercise too intensely without enough recovery and all it will do is add to your problems (including weight gain!).

If you are in an overstressed state from either life or your health improvement attempts, or both, then you really need to be mindful when implementing exercise. Don't get me wrong, you *should* do it. You just need to do it in a way that is honoring to the body. This is *not* the time to sign up for that boot camp or buy an "insane" DVD program. Again, listen to your body. You're looking for a restorative effect here—not to pile on and run yourself further into the ground.

Start off easy and with relatively low intensity. Sometimes going for a walk is all it takes to get the benefit of exercise without overtaxing yourself. By the end of the session you should feel comfortably fatigued. Don't be afraid to take days off either. Don't turn this into another stressful obsession where you feel like you can't miss a day. Again, listen to your body. If you start getting fatigued and you need more recovery time, then take it!

The only way you're going to stick with any exercise program is to do something you enjoy, or at least something you don't loathe. I firmly believe that how we feel about a given activity goes a long way toward determining how it affects us. If you are doing exercise you can't stand it is not going to be as beneficial as doing something you enjoy. If you detest walking on a treadmill, then don't do it. Go outside. Walk at the park. Go for a hike. You want to be able to say when you are finished, "I wouldn't mind doing that again tomorrow."

Lack of motivation can be a big clue that you may need more rest. If you have to regularly flex your willpower muscle in order to keep your self-imposed exercise commitment, you may be in need of a break. Err on the side of too much rest. When in doubt, sit it out.

Ideally you would do a little resistance work along with general cardio-type activities. You don't have to go to failure and scream on the last few reps but at least push your muscles and get a nice burn. You'll know you're doing it right because you'll get stronger and feel less soft and doughy. I also recommend you focus on strengthening your core as that has many real world benefits including helping with recurring low back and pelvic issues.

As you gain strength, endurance, and improved health

by exercising appropriately for your condition, by all means take it up a notch and continue to challenge yourself (without burning out!). You must, however, be ever vigilant and careful that you don't cross the line into overtraining or obsessive training. Ideally you are exercising to increase your health so you can go do something important with your life. It's a tool to help you thrive so that you can do something greater. Unless you're a professional athlete or make your living as a fitness model, it's not the point of life! Don't get sucked into the "must . . . do . . . more . . . !" trap where the next thing you know you're spending every waking moment trying to work up a sweat like you're Matthew Modine in *Vision Quest*.

Along with decreasing the stress load of the body by eating abundantly, getting plenty of sleep, resting as much as possible, proper hydration, and exercising appropriately, these changes will actually begin to *reverse* this condition, and encourage repair and restoration. In effect we've taken *causes* of ongoing stress and turned them into solutions.

Do the above recommendations cover *all* sources of physical and chemical stress? No way. I'm sure you can think of many other possible sources of stress, as can

I, but remember that the goal is to tackle this issue without turning into an obsessive, neurotic disaster. Simply browse some popular Internet health blogs and you can get so bogged down with minutiae that you could spend every hour of the day worrying that something out there is going to get you. All that does is generate more—you guessed it—stress. So don't sit around hand-wringing over the possibility that your Wi-Fi exposure could be altering your gut flora or that the leakage from your microwave is disabling your sperm tails. Just stick with the big stuff and you'll be okay.

I want to throw out a couple of more suggestions for what I have found to be the most useful and effective techniques for reducing stress on the body. These are not so much lifestyle changes as discussed above but rather practices you can incorporate to further help de-stress your system.

- » Chiropractic
- » Meditation
- » Yoga or Tai Chi

Chiropractic. Even though the public perception of chiropractic is that it's a conservative treatment for back pain, the real benefit of chiropractic care is that it reduces interference to the nervous system brought about by physical, chemical, and emotional stress. The only reason chiropractic is focused on the spine is because that's what houses your brain stem and spinal cord. As a chiropractor, I analyze the spine to determine the presence of vertebral subluxation, which is when a spinal bone misaligns causing interference to the nervous system. At this point it should be burned into your brain that when you decrease the stress load on the nervous system you set the stage for recovery and healing.

One of the tools we use to monitor and document nerve system interference and the presence of stress is called Heart Rate Variability (HRV), which is the beat to beat variability of the heart, and offers valuable information about autonomic nerve system function. HRV allows us to assess the overall level of autonomic nervous system function as well as the balance between sympathetic versus parasympathetic activity (the sympathetic response is the body's stress system).

What I have observed over the years, and that research has confirmed, is that reducing vertebral subluxation through adjusting the spine will commonly, in and of itself, lead to improvement in HRV readings. Simply put, regular chiropractic care reduces the stress load on the nervous system. Don't make the mistake many make in thinking that it's only useful for cranky backs. Many of my patients are asymptomatic and utilize chiropractic on a wellness basis as one of their primary strategies to keep stress levels to a minimum. You should too.

Meditation. Do I even need to explain this? Of course meditation is good for you and effective at bringing down stress levels. We all know that. The problem is that most of us find it difficult to do (especially in an overstressed state). If you don't wish to take ten years to learn how to meditate effectively, then there is a shortcut you might find useful. I call it Meditation: American Style.

There is very reasonably priced software you can download to create your own custom-made brain entrainment recordings for the purpose of effort-lessly getting your mind in a meditative state. By using sound technology that you listen to through headphones, you can dial up any brainwave pattern you choose including those for deep relaxation.

You simply put your headphones on, and lie down and hit "play" on your iPod or CD player. Close your eyes and listen to the pleasant sounds of a nature scene—for instance, rain falling or waves crashing on a beach—while the technology running in the background (entrainment) guides you into either alpha, beta, delta, or theta brainwaves, depending on what you want to accomplish. Sessions can be anywhere from ten minutes to over an hour.

I have personally used these and have taken HRV measurements before and after to test the immediate effect of the entrainment recordings and have seen impressive results, so I endorse this affordable, easy-to-use method of getting the benefits of meditation without the skill.

The software I prefer—another great tool to use in your de-stressing strategy—is called Neuro-Programmer and it's user-friendly, does a ton, and is very reasonably priced at under $100.

Yoga or Tai Chi. Both of these practices are known for their stress-reducing effects. I'll leave it to you to educate yourself on the details but I'm recommending them because they are easy on the body and are restorative in nature. Yes they are a form of exercise and you might even sweat a little, but they are still good for calming the stress response and improving you physically through the movements and poses.

So far you've got your diet squared away, you're hydrating properly, and you're getting plenty of sleep and rest as well as exercising appropriately for your situation. You're now going to a chiropractor as well as spending some time relaxing with brain entrainment recordings and maybe even taking a yoga or Tai Chi class now and then. An awesome start!

I've saved the biggest challenge for last. After the lifestyle decisions have been handled and you've stopped adding to the stress pile, you're left to tackle the biggest threat to your health and quality of life—emotional stress, the inner layer of the onion.

This is a huge topic and really *could* be the subject of an entire book. The fact that this is a get-to-the-point book prevents me from giving this topic as much attention as it deserves but let's at least throw some ideas out there to get you started. These suggestions come from my own experience as well as from the experience of working with thousands of patients over the years. Is this a complete list of *everything* you need to become mentally healthy, emotionally strong, and spiritually centered, thereby reducing your stress to a minimum? Of course not. I'm sure you'll be able to think of more to add but this should at least get you started.

One last thing. I understand and appreciate that some of the following suggestions will *not* be easy. In fact, a few of them will be some rather heavy lifting so if you need help with them, then by all means get help. I think counseling is great as long as you have an insightful, skilled counselor and not some hack that just wants to scribble on prescription pads. Sometimes an impartial view from someone you feel comfortable opening up to can give you some new insights and get you unstuck. It also is helpful to talk these issues through and get out of your head. So with that said, let's get to it.

In no particular order:

Be honest with yourself

Obviously if you're going to clean out the attic, you have to take inventory of what's going on up there. We all have a couple of dusty steamer trunks sitting up there full of stuff we should have thrown out or dealt with long ago. Identify those first. If you have some past trauma that you need to put to bed, then get to it. If you have an ongoing problem that you *know* is the primary source of stress in your life, acknowledge it. Don't live in denial. Get real with yourself even if it means irritating some old scars. If the ultimate goal is to arrive at a place of peace, then you can't pretend and distort reality. *Be honest with yourself.*

Take care of business

There are sources of stress we can do something about and sources of stress we can't do something about. For instance, if a huge source of stress is that you hate your job, then technically you can do something about it. You can quit. If your source of stress is because you're still torqued about how your mom treated you growing up but she's been dead for five years, well, there's not much you can do about that now. Identify your major stresses and decide which type they are because these are two different animals.

If you can do something about it, then address it. You can't go to a job you hate five days a week and expect to maintain a low-stress lifestyle. Not gonna happen. You *must* address it. Either quit, look for a new job, go back to school, learn a new skill, panhandle, *something*. Don't just accept your fate and let the life drain out of you. Take action. Likewise, if there's a stressful relationship that needs straightening out, then get to it. Once you claim victim status and accept it, you're toast. Don't be abused, taken advantage of, or bullied, and don't compromise your values. Assert yourself so you can live in peace.

If you can't do much about a stress because it's something from the past, then you're going to have to find a way to put it to bed. At its core, it means changing the way you think about it. I know, I know, easy to say. This is where you have to dig and fight for it though. Change the meaning of what happened. Find the good. Find the lesson (and no, "I learned from that experience that life sucks" is *not* an example of a helpful lesson). These kinds of stresses are tough no doubt, but if you can find a way to make peace, forgive, or otherwise let go, your life can be radically transformed.

Whether you need to address a current situation or relationship or change the way you think about the past, you need to step up and *take care of business.*

Give up the idea that you are in control

Sometimes we try to micromanage circumstances in a desperate attempt to control the outcome. Even with events that are obviously beyond our control we'll still exert mental energy trying to *will* them to go how we think they should go by worrying and fixating on them. This is exhausting, futile, and highly stressful. This is one of those areas where having a strong spiritual foundation is important. If you think everything in life is dependent on you, then I guess you'll be carrying around quite the burden. The reality, whether we like it or not, is that we control very little.

Letting go and giving up on the mirage of control is a great de-stressing thing to do. It takes faith, which is also a great de-stressing muscle to develop. Letting go of being the supervisor of the world will also delight those who have to deal with you on a regular basis, so everybody wins! Control what you can control (yourself to some degree) and *give up the idea that you are in control* of anything else.

Find your purpose

No one thrives while living an empty, pointless life. Finding a reason to live beyond staring at Instagram is essential to living a low-stress life. We need challenge. We need a reason to get up in the morning. We need to experience the positive stress of making a goal and reaching it. Sure we need to reduce the bad stress we've been discussing up to this point, but we also need to go after the good stuff!

I believe there is no coasting in life. You're either going upwards or you're rolling backwards. There is no staying the same. Unfortunately, unless you actively set your mind toward accomplishing something, the default setting seems to be doing just enough to survive, which upon closer inspection, is really rolling backwards.

Set goals. Make plans. Go for something. *Find your purpose.*

Focus on others

Notice I said focus on others, not compare yourself to others. This goes along with finding your purpose because I believe that as human beings we are at our best and most motivated when we're trying to help other people. It can't always be about you. While introspection and self-improvement are great to a degree, I think people today are taking it too far. If you're stuck in depression there's a good chance you've made your whole world about you. Turn your focus outward and do for others and you'll find things start to change.

While focusing on others is a great thing, comparing yourself to others is *so* not. As long as you compare yourself to others, you will always be left unsatisfied and wanting. There will always be people that have more stuff, have more fun, look better, smell better, and have thicker hair and more defined abs than you. And there's nothing peaceful about trying to keep up with the pretend world constructed by your friends' Facebook posts. It's the fast track to discontentment and depression, which incidentally, is very stressful. Compare you with *you*. Improve yourself in areas that matter. Yes, that means in areas *other* than your weight. Stop comparing yourself to others and start *focusing on others*.

Pursue contentment

This is the opposite of comparing yourself to others. Marketers love to keep you frothing at the mouth wondering if you have the latest and greatest. Don't get me wrong, stuff is nice and toys are fun, but when you can't be happy without more and more stuff, then you're going to a bad place. I can't imagine a scenario where we could be content and stressed at the same time. Come to think about it, contentment is almost a great *definition* of low stress.

The apostle Paul wrote, "I know what it is to be in need, and I know what it is to have plenty. I have learned the secret of being content in any and every situation, whether well fed or hungry, whether living in plenty or in want." Contentment is a learned trait and doesn't come naturally but it's a sign of spiritual maturity and something worth striving for. Paul thought it important enough to include in his ministry and his words made it into the Bible, so who are we to disagree? Pursue contentment.

Establish your boundaries and raise your standards

Boundaries are your rules on how you allow others to treat you; standards are the rules you set for yourself. Both are necessary. Don't establish clear boundaries and people will treat you however they wish. People can only mistreat us if we allow them. Sure someone may cross a line with you but if you've established boundaries, then you will have the strength to call them on it. Don't call them on it and it will become habit, resulting in hurt, resentment, and stress. Next thing you know you've become the family or neighborhood doormat. Not good. Decide for yourself what you will accept and what you won't accept from people.

Hold them to it. If someone in your world refuses to respect your boundaries, then show them the door. Trust me, it feels good.

Standards are equally important because they establish how you will in turn treat others (among other things). Standards are your code of conduct. It's much easier to call someone out for violating a boundary if you know you hold yourself to a high standard. It's healthy. High standards should come from a place of self-esteem not self-abuse. You should have high but reasonable expectations of yourself. It's about setting *high* standards, not *impossible* standards. If you don't have standards, or worse yet, if you violate the ones you have, it will result in damaged self-esteem, dysfunctional relationships, and increased stress. *Establish your boundaries and raise your standards.*

Pursue real relationships

A January 2016 study by Robin Dunbar, a professor of evolutionary psychology at Oxford University, reported that almost all Facebook "friends" are fake. What did they mean? Of the 150 Facebook friends the average user has, the researcher found that only fifteen could be counted as actual friends and only five as close friends. Yes, that means 90 percent of your Facebook "friends" really don't care what happens to you. The author goes on to state, "In practical terms, it may reflect the fact that real (as opposed to casual) relationships require at least occasional face-to-face interaction to maintain them."

Relationships can only go so far if they are lived through an electronic device. An important component of a low-stress lifestyle is relationships. Like, real ones. To have real ones you need to interact with people *in person*. It's amazing to me how many teenagers and young adults come into my office and cannot even have a basic conversation. I try to ask questions about their condition and all I get are one word answers, grunts, shoulder shrugs, and all-around awkwardness. I've been tempted to ask on more than one occasion, "Should I sit next to you and text you these questions?" Maybe then I'd get a coherent answer.

It's fairly well-established that social media and depression are linked. If you ask me, it's because it's a pretend world. Just like the study concluded, 90 percent of those friends really don't care what happens to you. It's a narcissistic playground where you compare your life with everyone else's highlight reel. It's not real. If real, face-to-face, emotionally invested relationships are meat and potatoes then social media relationships are a handful of marshmallows. Empty calories. Real relationships are health promoting and de-stressing, which is why you want to *pursue real relationships.*

Avoid codependency

Entire volumes have been written on this topic because it's so prevalent and damaging to our emotional health. It's defined as "excessive emotional or psychological reliance on a partner, typically a partner who requires support due to an illness or addiction." Another definition I prefer describes a codependent relationship as one person supporting or enabling another person's addiction, poor mental health, immaturity, irresponsibility, or underachievement. I like this definition because it expands the meaning past just enabling people with addiction.

This is getting more and more common because today's twenty-somethings, otherwise known as millennials, or as I prefer, Generation Selfie, have proven to be quite the incapable bunch. Harsh? Well apparently I'm not alone. A 2013 survey concluded that American millennials are arguably the most useless generation alive today. Ouch. This is resulting in record numbers of parents in their fifties having to carry their adult children because they can't function on their own.

Living in a codependent relationship is beyond stressful. It's flat-out destructive. This is one of those examples where well-established boundaries comes in very handy. If your well-being is dependent on how others behave or you've handed over the reins of your life to someone who doesn't know how to act, you're going to be up to your nostrils in stress. *That's why you must avoid codependency.*

Have realistic expectations

Agonizing over how you look is a very stressful way to live. When we compare ourselves to magazine covers, fitness models, and celebrities, then of course we're going to come up way short. Look, your body size is for the most part genetic and hereditary. There's a little you can do to influence it but for the most part, you look how you're going to look.

Many people have been sold on the idea that with hard work, the perfect diet, and unbreakable dedication, they can have the chiseled, speed bump abs that you see on the person selling the DVD workout collection.

Well the fact is that you probably can't. No matter what you do. If your parents are fat, your siblings are fat, your aunts, uncles, grandparents, and cousins are fat, then there's a good chance you're going to be fat too. So before you start putting all your eggs in the "I've got to look like Brad Pitt in Fight Club" basket please understand that it might not even be possible for you.

Unrealistic expectations have led to a *lot* of stress in a *lot* of people. Don't set yourself up for failure and a lifetime of anguish agonizing over your inability to get down to your "ideal" weight. It's really not worth it. Live as healthy as you can, live as low stress as you can, and see what happens. If you want to make improvements, start with subtle changes and monitor yourself to make sure they don't trigger a stress response. *It's all about subtle changes and realistic expectations.*

Disengage from media

Nothing foments internal strife like constant exposure to negativity. If you wanted to *induce* a stressful state the quickest way to do it would be to watch the news constantly with the endless killing, raping, and robbing stories intermixed with political pundits arguing back and forth. Realize that the goal of news stations and talk radio is to keep you watching and listening. They know if they can keep you all frothed up and emotional, they'll have a loyal customer. Don't fall for it.

The imprints and messages that your brain absorbs from media in a given day are powerful and play a huge role in your attitude, happiness levels, sense of hope, and overall mental health. The last thing we want to do is have our brains mulling over the negative news of the day while we're sleeping. We're supposed to de-stress during sleep not add more. Everybody knows the less time in front of the TV or computer, the better off we'll be. So give it a shot. Disengage from the drama of the world. Enjoy a quiet house or some music. Read a book. Guard what you let into your cranium via your senses. *Disengage from the media.*

Again, these are just a few suggestions on how to lower the levels of emotional stress in your life. If you do nothing but implement the ideas from this list that apply to you, I think you'll enjoy a much higher quality of life and you'll begin to turn the tide toward living a low-stress lifestyle.

Combine these emotional stress-reducing ideas with the previous suggestions on identifying and eliminating *self-imposed* stress causes and you've got yourself a real winner and a heck of a health strategy.

Put A Bow On It

I'm hopeful that you now have a clearer picture of how health is for the most part a function of how much, what kind, and in what way you handle stress, and how the choices you make concerning diet, exercise, and thinking go a long way toward either hurting or helping your cause.

I also expect that you can now see how your attempts at either regaining or optimizing your health and/or losing weight have possibly contributed to your health issues because of the massive stress burden they may have added.

The pursuit of health is a noble one, but it's one that can quickly get out from under you. Most people don't realize that all the tinkering and the "let's try this, let's try that" approach to health restoration can exact a heavy price and leave you wishing you had just left well enough alone. I'm confident though, if you apply the concepts in this book, that over time you will be able to pull yourself out of that hole and live a healthy life.

I made the statement at the beginning that this book is by a health professional who is trying to convince you to chill out with the health thing. I hope you will.

I've given you a very common sense approach to health and well-being that couldn't be easier to implement. It's completely free of any abusive practices, and it gives you permission to stop obsessing about your diet. You are now free to put your energy toward something useful.

Keep this little factoid in mind if you find yourself reverting back. Jack LaLanne, the famous and original US fitness guru who lived a life of pristine eating (including skipping the cake on his ninetieth birthday), daily exercising, juicing, and was the glowing example of all things health, passed away at the age of ninety-six. Pretty good, huh? What most people don't know, however, is that Jack had a brother. Norman. Norman LaLanne, who did *not* eat a pristine diet, did *not* exercise every day, reportedly hung out in his favorite barbecue joint, and said that the family always thought Jack was a little obsessive, recently died as well. He lived to be ninety-seven. Draw your own conclusion.

Now get out there, reduce your stress, be healthy, and enjoy your life—just don't forget to take some selfies.

WAIT . . . DON'T LEAVE ME!

I consider this book to be like a first date; granted, one where I did all the talking, and quite frankly, was a horrible listener. . . then again, you just sat there. You got to see a little of what I'm about and now it's time to decide if you want to see me again.

If the content of this book "scratched where you itched," then head on over to <u>healthnutrehab.com</u> and subscribe to my e-mail list. Because there's more where this came from, including an audio course based on this book that will be like a colonic for your brain.

So what did you think?

Thanks for spending a couple of hours with me. I'd be thrilled to know that you enjoyed the book and got something out of it, so I ask that you please take a moment and leave a review on Amazon. If I get enough favorable reviews, I may even be motivated to write another book!

Of course, if you thought the book sucked, then let's just keep that between us.